Sirtuins boosting! 25% less
(less calories is best)
reduction or fasting ? best.
(Resveratrol increases ↓ (every other day)

Effectiveness + activity)

Pr Louise Williams
(cards)

To the determined, curious and faithful

TABLE OF CONTENTS

INTRODUCTION

In 1990, I was a member of the University of Florida baseball team. Most days consisted of two and a half hours of practice under the Florida sun. You can imagine my regular appearance: a fully drenched uniform and skin striped with a distinguishing farmer's tan. The soaked-zebra look on the outside was funny enough, but something serious was taking place on the inside. A white salt-stained ring just above the bill of my ball cap was a sure sign of mineral depletion.

This gradual loss of critical minerals took a toll on my physiology. For many nights in a row when I would lie down to sleep, my heart would begin to speed up, slow down and skip beats. Was I having a heart attack? Was something seriously wrong with me? Ignorance of this frightening experience then created its own emotional anxiety, making the problem worse. The issue would come and go over the next year seemingly without any connection to my lifestyle. The symptoms ranged from mild and hardly noticeable to severe and scary.

It was at this time that my roommate, in search of his future career path, spoke of going to see his uncle, a chiropractor who did some "different" things. Little did he know that this seemingly random encounter would change my life. My roommate was right—Dr. Dugan was more than a chiropractor. He also practiced Applied Kinesiology (a cousin technique to Functional Bio-Analysis).

Throughout the years of his practice, Dr. Dugan developed a rapid evaluation that he performed on all his patients. It involved using the muscles as a semi-diagnostic tool. He explained to me that each muscle group connects to a related organ system: the deltoids to the lungs, the biceps to the stomach and so on. If a non-injured muscle did not stay "strong" under a steady pressure, the weakness signaled a potential problem.

On my first visit, he performed his assessment on me in the span of about eight minutes. My muscles easily resisted his pressure until he tested my right arm, specifically the subscapularis—a big muscle that starts on the underside of the shoulder blade, wraps around the ribs and attaches to the inside of the upper bone of the arm. It is one of the four muscles making up the rotator cuff. Mine had very little resistance. This of course was a shock to me. At the time I could decline press 300 pounds! By all outward assessments, I was a strong and healthy young man. Even so, Dr. Dugan could easily rotate my shoulder, and my subscapularis muscle could do nothing to stop him. He told me this muscle relates to the most active organ in the body, which happened to be another muscle—the heart.

To continue his exam, Dr. Dugan handed me two copper rods with electrical leads connected to a machine. It had a copper plate on top and some needle dials to measure electrical resistance. He had me hold one of the rods in each hand, and then he turned on the machine. The rods allowed a small electrical current to flow through my body. Next, Dr. Dugan placed different mineral supplements on the copper plate of the machine while keeping an eye on the dials. If my body didn't need the specific mineral on the plate, the dials didn't move.

Then something strange happened. The moment Dr. Dugan placed potassium on the copper plate, the dials sprang all the way from left to right. Something about potassium made a significant impact on the electrical flow through my body. What did that mean? To follow up on the reaction, Dr. Dugan removed the rods and instead, instructed me to simply hold the bottle of potassium in my left hand. He once again tested the subscapularis of my right arm. To my amazement, I now had full strength.

Based on my body's reactions, Dr. Dugan could tell I was functionally deficient in this important mineral. He prescribed the potassium as a supplement, and I faithfully obliged for the next three weeks, taking one or two potassium tablets per day. There was no great outward change. I already felt strong and healthy, but amazingly, I no longer had any heart issues. No speeding up or slowing down while at rest. Within days of taking the potassium, my heart palpitations stopped, and have not returned to this day.

The experience impressed me and raised many questions. How did my body know the bottle had potassium in it? How could my muscles change instantly to the presence of something outside my body? What about those connections between the muscles and the organs? Did muscle testing correlate with standard blood work or laboratory results? Could a doctor evaluate other things in the same way? Things like harmful chemicals, acupuncture meridians or even emotions? Through my studies in Applied Kinesiology, I found the answers to these and many other questions.

Muscle testing as a means to evaluate nutritional imbalances has come a long way in the 20 years since Dr. Dugan determined I had a potassium deficiency. Science has caught up as well, verifying much of what practitioners of Complementary and Alternative Medicine (CAM) have known all along. Research has discovered many of the nutrients critical to neurological and immune system function. This knowledge means that if a doctor were to know which systems were out of balance, he could then use FBA to discover which nutrients the body needed to restore balance, or homeostasis. This happens every day in the offices of FBA physicians.

Personally, I have used this approach to help thousands of patients with some of the most common, challenging and expensive illnesses affecting the civilized population today: depression, diabetes, digestive issues, heart disease, hormonal imbalances, hypoglycemia, metabolic issues, migraines and many forms of pain. Even significant and frightening conditions such as auto-immune disorders can be helped markedly or go into remission altogether with FBA. Many of the common ailments FBA regularly resolves, are discussed throughout the pages of *Hope for Health*.

If used generally, FBA would revolutionize health care as we know it, making doctors more preventative and patients more proactive. The consequences would result in greatly reduced costs and a significant reduction in chronic illness. But there is so much more.

Hope for Health is a book about correcting functional illness—the place between optimal health and recognizable disease. Functional illness is the realm where traditional medicine has few answers, but where the needs are the greatest. It is the reason why exercising no longer means losing weight. It is why eating healthy no longer rebuilds tissues or restores nutrient levels. It is why fatigue and pain are the greatest complaints for those who see a doctor. It is why sleep is interrupted when stress has long passed. It is why so many women have PMS, hypoglycemia, poor thyroid function and struggle with infertility. It is where you are right now.

Before delving into the mechanics of Functional Bio-Analysis and its benefits for helping achieve optimal health, it is important to get an overview of the processes that promote illness, disease, and aging. Just as important, is knowing how these processes fit together. Which are the most common? The most detrimental? What are the inward and outward signs? In other words, what are the common pitfalls to avoid and the steps to take to encourage and maintain health? This knowledge is cutting-edge and motivating, and since these topics are of greatest interest to most, they are presented in the first two chapters, *Health & The Stress Threshold* and *The Fountain of Youth & Anti-Aging?*

As you are about to learn, the human body is a metabolic maze, vulnerable to attack on many fronts. There is no such thing as a condition in isolation. Every complaint has multiple potential causes. Pinpointing the disrupted areas is what FBA does best. Correcting those areas with what the body needs most is how miracles happen. It means patients begin to get better. It means discouragement begins to dissipate. It means there is hope for health.

HEALTH & THE STRESS THRESHOLD

*There are two educations. One should teach us how to make a living
and the other how to live.*
John Adams, Second President of the United States

It was always possible for humans to fly. The laws of physics didn't change once the Wright brothers invented the airplane. Orville and Wilbur simply made use of air's natural properties, something that was always present. True, they first needed a familiarity with a particular base of knowledge to see what was possible. Health is much the same way. Being healthy requires an understanding of some fundamental laws of the body—laws that most never knew existed, although they rely on them every day. This understanding must start with a good working definition of health – a word which has been hijacked to mean anything from feeling good to looking good to simply making it to a certain age.

Is health how a person feels? Most people believe they are healthy. According to the National Health Interview Survey (NHIS), respondents were asked to assess their own health and that of family members living in the same household as excellent, very good, good, fair, or poor. The percentage of people who believed they had excellent or very good health was 65.6 percent in 2010.[1]

It is much the same around the world. The results of the Second European Quality of Life Survey mimicked those found in the United States, with roughly two-thirds of people in the UK believing they were in "good" or "very good" health.[2] Is it possible that two-thirds of the people walking down Main Street, through the grocery store, or in the mall are in excellent or very good health? The NHIS data did come closer to reflecting reality among those over 65. By then, only 41.7 percent of respondents believed they had excellent or very good health.[3]

Is health the absence of disease? Perhaps those above had no diagnosed disease at the time of their survey, so they considered themselves healthy. Maybe they just need to wait a few more years. Diseases overall, including cancer, heart disease, and obesity, continue to rise.[4] At the same time, mental disorders are advancing to the top of the global list of diseases. Estimates predict depression will become the second most common disease by the year 2020.[5]

Is health a long life? The average life expectancy in industrialized countries continues to rise.[6] In 2010, life expectancy for men was around 77 years and for women 81 years. To the credit of traditional medicine, people appear to suffer from more diseases but live through them, or at least with them. However, this brings up the question of quality of life. Is someone who lives to 85 years old with the effort of multiple medications, surgeries, and significant physical limitations considered healthy?

The World Health Organization (WHO) defines health as, "*A state of complete physical, mental and social well-being and not merely the absence of disease or infirmity.*" This sounds nice. Unfortunately, the WHO definition is nebulous and lofty and could use a bit of earth under its toes.

What is critical to, and missing from, the definition of health is the category of functional illness. Free falling from perfect health to disease is not the norm. Long before disease was in the picture, functional illness was visible, perhaps even in the foreground. Consequently, to properly gage one's current health, functional illness must be assessed, subjective bias must be reduced and a final element should be considered: quality of life. All of these factors are the framework of the *Functional Health Assessment.*

With a functional illness, a person will have symptoms (sometimes debilitating ones), but his or her life is not in immediate danger. The illness is a signal by the body that something is wrong, out-of-balance. Headaches, insomnia, indigestion, joint pain, hormonal imbalances, and dozens of other "normal" complaints are all common signs of functional problems. These conditions and many others are warnings that health is in jeopardy. They are also chinks in the armor of modern medicine, since medications and surgery in these cases do no good, are unnecessary, or create a slew of harmful side effects that are worse than the original condition. The good news is that functional illness is in the realm of Complementary and Alternative Medicine, and the specialty of Functional Bio-Analysis.

Looking at the graph below, health is the region beneath the dotted line. It is distinct from both functional illness and disease. The demarcation in

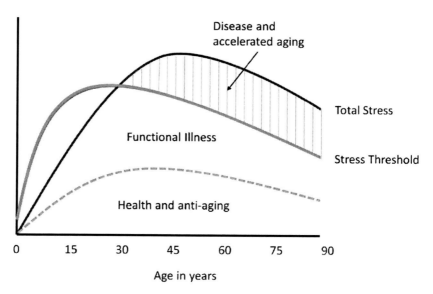

The Stress Threshold

between functional illness and disease is the *Stress Threshold*. Exceeding this threshold is something people never want to do. Everyone's threshold is unique, variable, and based upon genetic strengths and the total amount of accumulated stress. The definition of stress is more than just emotional unrest. Stress is also structural trauma or chemical deficiencies and toxicities, which each have their own detrimental effect on health.

Stress is a natural part of life. Without it, people could not mature emotionally or physically. The dilemma occurs when the stresses of life overwhelm the body's ability to cope. In fact, too much stress produces adverse effects in roughly 43 percent of all adults and has a relationship in some way or another to 75 - 90 percent of all medical visits. Stress also contributes to chronic illnesses, such as cardiovascular disease, diabetes, osteoporosis, gastrointestinal disorders, obesity, cancer, anxiety, and depression.[78] Often, just the thought of a stressful event is enough to cause an increased heart rate, perspiration, or in severe cases, panic attacks.

Short-term stress, if severe enough, may generate functional imbalances and push a person toward the stress threshold, whereas long-term stress lowers the stress threshold entirely. This is why people who have managed ongoing ailments for years are easily pushed over the brink physically and emotionally—their reserves and the stress threshold itself are near the bottom.

For example, two similar men were healthy, each having low total stress and a high stress threshold at the beginning of the year. The first man had a good year: No one in his family died, he had a stable job, and all close relationships remained intact. The second man started the year with an analogous profile, but things quickly changed: doctors diagnosed a good friend with cancer, a competitor bought his corporation, putting his job in jeopardy, and the downturned economy soured several investments. On top of this, the office building where he worked experienced a major water leak and later tested positive for high levels of airborne mold. After one year's time, two things happened to the second man. First, he rapidly moved toward his stress threshold. The results of this most likely included functional imbalances, such as insomnia, irritability, digestive complaints, and even perhaps, depression. Second, the ongoing nature of his stress lowered the overall threshold entirely, setting him up for even worse problems in the future.

To their credit, complementary doctors of all sorts recognize that nearly all dysfunction is the result of multiple factors, present within multiple layers. This means that dysfunction has more than one cause. Physical conditions like fibromyalgia, chronic fatigue syndrome, autoimmune issues, and congenital disorders, are amalgamations of multiple imbalances.[9] [10] [11] [12] However, *all* functional illness is multi-layered and the problem gets worse. Once present, functional illness initiates a self-perpetuating cycle that simultaneously affects the emotional, structural, and metabolic planes.

When faced with this dilemma, alternative medicine doctors may employ natural strategies, such as detoxification protocols, food allergy elimination, and psychological therapies, in the hopes of removing enough total stress from the ailing body to allow for an increased quality of life. Often, these approaches are helpful to some degree but not for everyone in every circumstance. A greater understanding of the causes, called the pathophysiology, and more therapeutic specificity is required.

FUNCTIONAL ILLNESS – A THREE HEADED MONSTER

Conditions with multiple imbalances do have common characteristics. The three systems responsible for most functional illness are the same three systems that manifest most often with Functional Bio-Analysis. They are defined by the acronym HIT: Hormonal dysregulation, immune system dysfunction, and toxicity.

Hormonal dysregulation can refer to any hormonal problem, but it most often means abnormal insulin from a blood sugar imbalance and abnormal cortisol from the stress response. Immune system dysfunction means all kinds of autoimmunity and inflammation. Finally, toxicity refers to the bombardment of environmental and food-based chemicals that inundate the human body.

Three of the four sections in the Functional Health Assessment below are arranged based on HIT. Any category of HIT, once ignited, is a catalyst, kick starting the other two. To put it mildly, ongoing HIT is a threat to a person's current quality of life. HIT sets individuals up for disease by applying downward pressure on the cells, which are the home of the genes.

With the consideration of functional illness, a simple definition of health begins to emerge. **Health is the state of being far below one's stress threshold.** Unhealthy would be just the opposite: near to or beyond the threshold. Although no lab test can pinpoint where one's stress threshold may be, tracking the signs and symptoms of functional illness and quality of life makes assessing one's health much easier. The more functional problems present at any one time, the worse the state of health and the greater the risk for future disease.

TEST YOUR STRESS THRESHOLD

Before a person can get to where he is going, it is essential to know where he is. The test on the next page, called a *Functional Health Assessment*, helps people to quantify their current health level and generate a baseline. The totals from each section are added together, converted into a grade value and then superimposed on the *Stress Threshold* graph. Individuals should repeat this test every six weeks as they employ the strategies in *Hope for Health* or follow the recommendations of an FBA practitioner.

To complete the test, circle the number to the right of each question, with 0 being no severity to 5 being the highest severity.

SECTION I – HORMONAL ASSESSMENT

Acne on face?	0	1	2	3	4	5
Always hungry?	0	1	2	3	4	5
Anxious for no apparent reason?	0	1	2	3	4	5
Crave breads?	0	1	2	3	4	5
Crave salt?	0	1	2	3	4	5
Crave sweets after meals?	0	1	2	3	4	5
Crave sweets throughout the day?	0	1	2	3	4	5
Depression during monthly period?	0	1	2	3	4	5
Difficulty urinating?	0	1	2	3	4	5
Dizziness upon standing?	0	1	2	3	4	5
Emotional outbursts?	0	1	2	3	4	5
Energy drops in the afternoon?	0	1	2	3	4	5
Facial hair growth?	0	1	2	3	4	5
Have or had asthma?	0	1	2	3	4	5
Headaches around menstrual cycle?	0	1	2	3	4	5
Headaches in the morning?	0	1	2	3	4	5
Headaches with exertion or stress?	0	1	2	3	4	5
Hot flashes?	0	1	2	3	4	5
Irregular monthly cycles?	0	1	2	3	4	5
Irritable or lightheaded between meals?	0	1	2	3	4	5
Less than 8 hours of sleep per night?	0	1	2	3	4	5
Light bothers eyes (always wear sunglasses)?	0	1	2	3	4	5
Loss of sexual desire?	0	1	2	3	4	5
Loss of sexual performance?	0	1	2	3	4	5

Low blood pressure?	0 1 2 3 4 5
Menstrual cramping?	0 1 2 3 4 5
Night sweats?	0 1 2 3 4 5
Outer third of eyebrow thinning?	0 1 2 3 4 5
Poor night vision?	0 1 2 3 4 5
Prostatitis or vaginitis (itching)?	0 1 2 3 4 5
Restless legs?	0 1 2 3 4 5
Shaky or lightheaded if you miss a meal?	0 1 2 3 4 5
Shortness of breath?	0 1 2 3 4 5
Trouble losing weight even with exercise?	0 1 2 3 4 5
Trouble staying asleep?	0 1 2 3 4 5
Vaginal yeast infections?	0 1 2 3 4 5
Vision changes throughout the day?	0 1 2 3 4 5
Weight gain without diet or lifestyle changes?	0 1 2 3 4 5
Weight loss without diet or lifestyle changes?	0 1 2 3 4 5

SECTION II – IMMUNE & INFLAMMATORY ASSESSMENT

Abdominal bloating after eating?	0 1 2 3 4 5
Can't remember the names of people I just met?	0 1 2 3 4 5
Can't turn off my mind when it is time to relax?	0 1 2 3 4 5
Chest pains?	0 1 2 3 4 5
Cold hands or feet?	0 1 2 3 4 5
Cold sores?	0 1 2 3 4 5
Colitis?	0 1 2 3 4 5
Does caffeine make you feel bad?	0 1 2 3 4 5
Does caffeine make you feel good?	0 1 2 3 4 5
Does sugar make you feel bad?	0 1 2 3 4 5
Does sugar make you feel good?	0 1 2 3 4 5
Dry skin?	0 1 2 3 4 5
Excessive hair loss?	0 1 2 3 4 5
Fatigue?	0 1 2 3 4 5
Feel worse in humid, damp, or moldy places?	0 1 2 3 4 5
Fungus under finger or toenails?	0 1 2 3 4 5
Gluten intolerance?	0 1 2 3 4 5
Growing pains as a child?	0 1 2 3 4 5
Have a feeling of dependency on others?	0 1 2 3 4 5
Have a feeling of dread or impending doom?	0 1 2 3 4 5
Have a hard time finishing tasks?	0 1 2 3 4 5
Have difficulty calculating numbers?	0 1 2 3 4 5
Heartburn?	0 1 2 3 4 5

Hemorrhoids?	0	1	2	3	4	5
High blood pressure?	0	1	2	3	4	5
Hives?	0	1	2	3	4	5
Loss of long-term memory?	0	1	2	3	4	5
Loss of short-term memory?	0	1	2	3	4	5
Loss of smell?	0	1	2	3	4	5
Loss of taste?	0	1	2	3	4	5
Lower back pain?	0	1	2	3	4	5
Mind often wanders even while doing important things?	0	1	2	3	4	5
Nails are weak?	0	1	2	3	4	5
Nails have ridges?	0	1	2	3	4	5
Nails peel?	0	1	2	3	4	5
Nasal or sinus congestion?	0	1	2	3	4	5
Neck pain?	0	1	2	3	4	5
Numbness in toes not related to injury?	0	1	2	3	4	5
Pins and needles in arms?	0	1	2	3	4	5
Regular headaches?	0	1	2	3	4	5
Ringing in ears?	0	1	2	3	4	5
Skin wrinkling rapidly?	0	1	2	3	4	5
Slow healing sores?	0	1	2	3	4	5
Spider veins?	0	1	2	3	4	5
Spoon-shaped indented nails?	0	1	2	3	4	5
Stomach ulcers?	0	1	2	3	4	5
Sweat often?	0	1	2	3	4	5
Swelling in ankles?	0	1	2	3	4	5
Varicose veins?	0	1	2	3	4	5
Visual problems?	0	1	2	3	4	5

SECTION III – TOXICITY ASSESSMENT

Abdominal pain?	0	1	2	3	4	5
Acne on back or legs?	0	1	2	3	4	5
Arthritis?	0	1	2	3	4	5
Bad breath?	0	1	2	3	4	5
Breast tenderness during menstrual cycle?	0	1	2	3	4	5
Burning pains in joints, muscles, or skin?	0	1	2	3	4	5
Coated or fuzzy tongue?	0	1	2	3	4	5
Crave alcoholic beverages?	0	1	2	3	4	5
Diarrhea after a fatty meal?	0	1	2	3	4	5
Do chemical smells or exposure cause symptoms?	0	1	2	3	4	5
Dread getting up each day to experience life?	0	1	2	3	4	5
Eczema?	0	1	2	3	4	5
Food allergies?	0	1	2	3	4	5
Frequent skin rashes?	0	1	2	3	4	5
Gallstones?	0	1	2	3	4	5
Handle problems effectively?	0	1	2	3	4	5
High cholesterol?	0	1	2	3	4	5
History of Hepatitis?	0	1	2	3	4	5
I do not have hobbies and interests that I actively engage in?	0	1	2	3	4	5
Leg cramps?	0	1	2	3	4	5
Muscle tenderness without exercise?	0	1	2	3	4	5
Often wake up between 2 and 4 a.m.?	0	1	2	3	4	5
Pain or swelling in joints?	0	1	2	3	4	5

Pet allergies?	0	1	2	3	4	5
Psoriasis?	0	1	2	3	4	5
Regular constipation?	0	1	2	3	4	5
Regular diarrhea?	0	1	2	3	4	5
Regular digestive complaints?	0	1	2	3	4	5
Sore joints with exercise?	0	1	2	3	4	5
Tobacco smoke is very offensive?	0	1	2	3	4	5
Trouble falling asleep?	0	1	2	3	4	5

SECTION IV – VITALITY ASSESSMENT

This final section contains questions related to circumstances that may prevent or slow down the recovery of health. Changes in lifestyle may modify or eliminate many of them. Others are circumstances in the past that no longer apply or may be uncontrollable, such as family history.

20+ pounds overweight?	0 1 2 3 4 5
Airline pilot?	0 1 2 3 4 5
Alcohol consumption per week?	0 1 2 3 4 5
Antibiotic use (this year or more than three times in the last ten years)?	0 1 2 3 4 5
Average level of stress for the last three months?	0 1 2 3 4 5
Average level of stress over the last year?	0 1 2 3 4 5
Average level of stress throughout your life?	0 1 2 3 4 5
Currently level of stress?	0 1 2 3 4 5
Drink less than 4 glasses of water per day?	0 1 2 3 4 5
Eat less than 1 piece of fruit and 2 vegetable servings per day?	0 1 2 3 4 5
Eat out more than twice per week?	0 1 2 3 4 5
Family history of cancer?	0 1 2 3 4 5
Family history of diabetes?	0 1 2 3 4 5
Family history of heart disease?	0 1 2 3 4 5
Family history of mental illness?	0 1 2 3 4 5
Family history of stroke?	0 1 2 3 4 5
Feel disinterested with former hobbies?	0 1 2 3 4 5
Feel hopeless about my situation?	0 1 2 3 4 5

Feel little compassion for others?	0	1	2	3	4	5
Feel that I have no purpose?	0	1	2	3	4	5
Feel that life is meaningless?	0	1	2	3	4	5
Feel uninterested with life?	0	1	2	3	4	5
Have used oral steroids?	0	1	2	3	4	5
Hospitalized for a non-emergency in the last 12 months?	0	1	2	3	4	5
Hospitalized for a non-traumatic emergency in the last 12 months?	0	1	2	3	4	5
Little or no exercise?	0	1	2	3	4	5
Major lifestyle change (divorce, loss of job, relocation, death of loved one, etc.)?	0	1	2	3	4	5
Often eating meals after 8 p.m.?	0	1	2	3	4	5
Oral contraceptive use (past or present)?	0	1	2	3	4	5
Serious accident or injury in your lifetime?	0	1	2	3	4	5
Sick about once per year?	0	1	2	3	4	5
Sick more than once per year?	0	1	2	3	4	5
Smoker?	0	1	2	3	4	5
Sun exposure less than 15 min. per day?	0	1	2	3	4	5
Surgery (other)?	0	1	2	3	4	5
Surgery as a result of trauma?	0	1	2	3	4	5
Surgery on a joint?	0	1	2	3	4	5
Surgery on internal organs?	0	1	2	3	4	5
Taking more than 2 medications?	0	1	2	3	4	5
Under frequent high stress?	0	1	2	3	4	5
Work with computers daily?	0	1	2	3	4	5

ANALYZING THE RESULTS

To calculate an overall health grade, add up the total of the circled answers for each section. Then, add the total for the first three sections together to make one score. Section IV will be computed separately. The total score from a given section is better than just counting all the questions with high scores. From a functional perspective, multiple sets of low scores are equivalent to a few sets of high scores. Once you have the sections added together as instructed, find the corresponding grade on the chart below.

GRADE	SECTIONS I-III TOTAL SCORE	SECTION IV VITALITY	COMMENTS
A	<50	<40	Few functional complaints with high vitality
B	<70	<50	Low to moderate functional complaints with good vitality
C	<90	<60	Moderate functional complaints with moderate vitality
D	<110	<70	Elevated functional complaints with low moderate vitality
F	>130	>80	Excessive functional complaints with low vitality

Now, match the grade with the corresponding letter on the *Stress Threshold* graph below. This is your current placement.

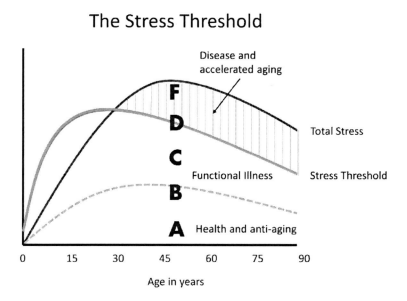

Figure 1: Grading the Stress Threshold

The golden rule of prevention states that the best time to fix a problem is before it ever happens. However, human nature being what it is, most people only seek help from an FBA practitioner after first amassing dozens of functional problems, or the equivalent of a grade C, D, or F. If this is true in your case, do not worry. Functional Bio-Analysis brings health to those unhelped and those long dismissed by their medical doctors. The knowledge gained through *Hope for Health* is a great place to start.

Having an understanding of functional illness, it is now time to investigate its origins and the mechanisms that allow it to perpetuate. In other words, it is time to look at how the wheels fell off the cart. Knowing this information will be of service for both health rejuvenation and longevity.

THE FOUNTAIN OF YOUTH & ANTI-AGING?

Since well before Ponce de León scoured the New World looking for the Fountain of Youth, humans have been intensely interested in immortality. As many ancient civilizations observed, health and longevity correlate with diet, nutrition, and lifestyle practices. Nothing has changed. Today, researchers and physicians can demonstrate scientifically that overconsumption of the wrong food types and poor lifestyle choices lead directly to genetic damage and disease. The result of this ancient wisdom and current scientific corroboration is the emergence of a field of study called Nutritional Genomics. None of this is too surprising. People are sophisticated enough to realize that a good diet, exercise, and avoiding stress are essential to health. Yet, none of these necessarily guarantees longevity. So, is there a magic bullet for aging?

In order to answer this question, we must first answer another. What exactly is aging? What is the mechanism? The answer: aging is imperfect cell replication. Think of it this way. If a perfect cell could replicate itself perfectly, the result would be another perfect cell. If this process happened continuously and indefinitely the outcome would be anti-aging, or natural immortality. A quick look at the wedding album or the high school yearbook is proof that this idyllic state has yet to occur.

If one were able to find a fountain or herb or fruit to increase longevity, what would it do to prevent disease and halt the aging process? Would it grow new cells? Would it balance all hormones? Would it prevent free radical assault? In other words, is there a common characteristic—an origin of illness, if you will, between functional imbalances, diseases, and even aging, that if addressed would help correct and prevent all three? The short answer appears to be yes.

TELOMERES & EPIGENETICS

All cells have within them a biological clock that determines the maximum number of times they can divide. Cell death is called senescence[13] and takes place after about 70 cell divisions in young cells and far less in older cells.[14] However, cells rarely reach natural senescence. Instead, they often die long before their time for another reason: failure to fully replicate DNA.

Four types of small building blocks called nucleotides combine to make DNA. Arranging these nucleotides properly is the essence of DNA replication during cell division. DNA is a double helical organization of nearly one billion nucleotides. In order for DNA to copy itself, it must first "unzip." The two separated halves then must recreate their missing side. If all goes well, the end result is a perfect copy of the original "parent" DNA. However, ending up with a perfect DNA copy is often a less than perfect process.

As nucleotides are added to an unzipped side, mismatches are consistently generated. Called single nucleotide polymorphisms or SNPs (pronounced "Snips"), these bad sections of DNA must be discarded and replaced. Each cell is more than prepared for this contingency by keeping plenty of spare parts (nucleotides) nearby. All DNA contain redundant, long, and repetitive sequences of nucleotides. These spare parts, called telomeres, are the key to health rejuvenation and anti-aging.

Visualized as an aglet, the little plastic part on the end of a shoelace, telomeres are located at the tips of the DNA strand.[15] Cells with long telomeres flawlessly replicate their DNA. Those with short telomeres do not. A strong correlation exists between short telomeres and disease. Every time a cell divides, telomeres become shorter, genetic material becomes less stable, and diseases are likely to increase.[16] [17] [18]

Embryonic cells start off with telomeres around 15,000 nucleotides long. At birth, the telomeres have decreased in length to approximately 10,000 nucleotides. They continue to shorten throughout a person's lifetime to an average of about 5,000 nucleotides. Below this number, cells are unable to divide further, and the end result is death from old age. That is, unless telomeres were able to lengthen again.[19] Researchers know there must be a way to regrow or prevent telomeres from shortening, since in some cells this is already taking place.

The reproductive cells, sperm and egg, do not have shortened telomeres no matter how old they may be. The reason for this phenomenon is an enzyme called telomerase. In laboratory testing, cells with plenty of telomerase do not die and do not manifest disease.[20] [21] What is interesting is that all cells have the potential to manufacture this mysterious enzyme, but they do not. Like a cell phone resting quietly on the nightstand until its number is dialed, telomerase genes within every cell await the proper environmental signal before being prompted to action. Whatever turns on telomerase, prevents biological aging.

As one might expect, the pharmaceutical industry is working enthusiastically to develop effective drugs designed to lengthen telomeres by increasing telomerase activity within the cells. The research holds promise but is still many decades off. There is no need to despair or to rush out and purchase a cryogenic chamber in the hopes of being unfrozen and scientifically resurrected at some point in the Orwellian future. Anti-aging can begin immediately by putting into practice those things already known to increase telomerase activity and by avoiding those that don't.

Stress on a cell means more frequent division and a faster road to senescence. Lifestyle factors that stimulate disease processes will also shorten telomeres and reduce telomerase activity. Common factors include psychological stress,[22] [23] [24] oxidation,[25] [26] [27] [28] and blood sugar imbalances.[29] [30] At the same time, lifestyle factors known to promote health, such as aerobic exercise,[31] [32] [33] lengthen telomeres. On the whole, a person can encourage telomerase activity with an anti-inflammatory diet, certain nutritional supplements, regular moderate exercise, and stress management.[34] These well-known remedies effect genetic expression from outside the cell, having what cellular biologists call an epigenetic influence.

Epigenetics

How genes express themselves determines everything about the body, including how it looks, functions, and heals. Diseases, as well, can be the result of gene expression, or the lack thereof. For many years, scientists believed that bad genes were the reason for *all* diseases. If a person had a given disease-gene, she was in trouble. If she did not, then the coast was clear. But, not all women with the gene for breast cancer actually developed the disease. Some women are able to keep the gene from turning on.

The Human Genome Project set out to catalog all the different genes within the body. Expecting to find 120,000 or more genes located within the twenty-three pairs of human chromosomes, scientists were more than surprised to discover only around one fifth of that number. This shocking revelation made it clear: Genes were not the exclusive determinant of destiny. There were simply not enough of them to account for all the potential traits and diseases.

Still reeling from this earthquake under the microscope, classical genetic engineers were about to be hit with a tsunami. Science now knows that a single gene has not one but around 30,000 potential forms of expression.[35] As it turns out, all manner of outer environmental influences, such as stress, nutrition, exercise and even thoughts have a profound effect on what the gene does and when it does it. All of this means that genes, as was thought for decades, are not deterministic, but are instead a set of possibilities. These phenomena and their new realities are the realm of epigenetics. As epigenetic influences lay siege to the body, functional imbalances appear, manifesting as any of the symptoms listed on the *Functional Health Assessment.*

Of all the extra-cellular factors that influence genetic expression the ones that are garnering the most attention by epigeneticists are the emotions. Every thought and feeling produces thousands of chemical components, which have the potential to influence genes, turning them "on" or "off." Negative emotional states and their detrimental effect on health are easily understood, but if mere thoughts have the potential to alter genetic expression, then emotional health instantly becomes a top priority. A discussion of some of the emotional techniques used by FBA practitioners to restore well-being is presented in Appendix A.

Protecting the cells from epigenetic influences on the outside is a path of prevention, rejuvenation and vitality. However, protecting the cells on the inside slows down biological aging and is therefore the road to longevity. **The origin of both aging and illness begins with inflammation inside the cell itself.**

INFLAMMATION & FREE RADICALS

Inflammation is the recognized process that occurs after the onset of an injury or an infection. Anything red, swollen, and painful on the outside is probably inflammation. Joint aches and muscular pains resulting from a viral or bacterial illness are common, as well. The inflammatory process, initiated and controlled by the immune system, is essential for tissue repair and healing and to eliminate foreign organisms. Like a posse sent out to round up a gang of horse thieves, the immune system sends forth deputized chemicals for a select purpose. Macrophages, eosinophils, basophils, and neutrophils gallop out of town in search of justice. To keep the sometimes heavy-handed chemicals from doing more harm than good, strong anti-inflammatory agents, such as cortisol from the adrenal glands, travel alongside and prevent the inflammatory posse from taking the law into its own hands. Without this stopgap, immune-based diseases like asthma, rheumatoid arthritis, and Multiple Sclerosis may ultimately occur.

The forms of inflammation mentioned so far originate outside of the cell itself. Outside inflammation is essential for combating the injuries or organisms that threaten health and function. However, the efficiency of outside-cell processes is dependent upon proper function inside the cells.

The cell is a miniature version of the entire body. It contains all the major processes of the body and has the functional equivalent of a brain, organs, a nervous system, a reproductive system, and even an immune system. Before a disease or dysfunction can ever manifest in the body, inflammation is first brewing in the cells. In other words, as the cell goes, so the body goes. Therapies and techniques that best address cellular inflammation are the most desirable and effective for promoting health and longevity. The figure below shows the four main areas where inflammation can occur.

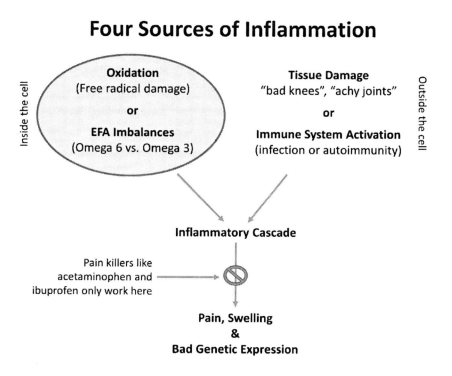

Four Sources of Inflammation

No matter the source of the inflammation, painkillers like acetaminophen, ibuprofen, and naproxen work to stop the process after it has long been underway. These over-the-counter medications are in a class called nonsteroidal anti-inflammatory drugs (NSAIDS). Using NSAIDS for pain management due to an occasional injury, like a sprained ankle, poses no detrimental effect. However, daily use of NSAIDS for body aches and pains or to manage arthritis indicates a deeper level of dysfunction within the cells themselves, one that may in fact turn deadly. In the United States, overuse of NSAIDS accounts for around 16,000 deaths annually.[36] [37] A holistic approach would attempt to prevent inflammation in the first place. Igniting the inflammatory flame can result from several sparks. Smothering these embers is the hope of both health and anti-aging.

Free Radicals

The essential elements for life are in many cases the same things that facilitate disease and aging. Everything must be in its designed balance. Sunlight is essential for maintaining hormonal balance by initiating the production of vitamin D and encouraging natural biorhythms, but too much leads to disease of the skin. Inflammation heals damaged tissues and rids bodies of foreign invaders, but too much destroys healthy tissues and leads to conditions like arthritis and eczema . Oxygen is critical for life, but too much damages DNA and promotes poor genetic expression. In this last case, oxygen, when in contact with certain molecules, alters their shape. This is oxygenation, and it is the source of most free radicals.

A free radical is the leftover molecule after oxygen or another substance has stolen away an electron. Like an obnoxious nine-year-old zinged up on sugar whose favorite toy has gone missing, this rogue molecule is an unstable troublemaker and will remain so until it gets its electron back. There are many forms of free radicals. The ones caused by oxidation are called reactive oxygen species (ROS). These chemicals are produced under normal circumstances inside cells every time oxygen is present, which is nearly always. Cleary, oxygen is essential, but its residue – oxidation - is the precursor of aging and the pathway to disease.

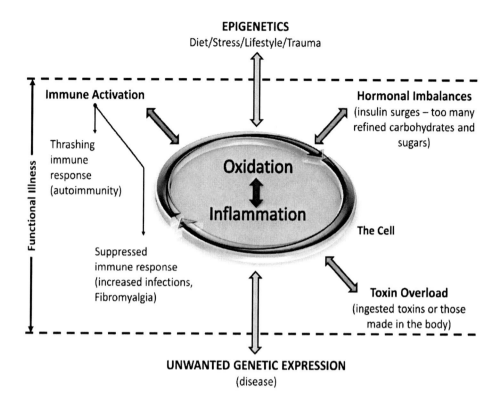

EPIGENETICS
Diet/Stress/Lifestyle/Trauma

Immune Activation

Thrashing immune response (autoimmunity)

Suppressed immune response (increased infections, Fibromyalgia)

Functional Illness

Oxidation
Inflammation

The Cell

Hormonal Imbalances
(insulin surges – too many refined carbohydrates and sugars)

Toxin Overload
(ingested toxins or those made in the body)

UNWANTED GENETIC EXPRESSION
(disease)

Oxidation promotes aging since the free radicals produced do damage to the DNA.[38] Like a springtime hailstorm in Kansas, it is estimated that the DNA must withstand up to 100,000 oxidative hits per day.[39] This bombardment changes the structure of DNA, damaging pieces of the gene itself, resulting in a polymorphism. Free radical inflammation makes SNP repair difficult and results in junk DNA, which shortens telomeres and further increases the potential for disease.

Despite their frequency and intensity, free radicals are not a problem, as long as the body can neutralize them. This is the job of antioxidants. Antioxidants can be any of a number of compounds, including vitamins, minerals, and botanicals. Vitamins A, C, and E, zinc, and selenium are common ones. Other categories of antioxidants, such as carotenoids, flavonoids, and isoflavones, are less familiar but just as vital. All these come from natural foods (ones without wrappers). Regular ingestion of fruits and vegetables increases stored antioxidants. If the body has depleted antioxidant reserves, free radicals can significantly injure cells and leave DNA unrepaired. In this state, even breathing oxygen-filled air is damaging.

The army of antioxidants inside and outside the cells constantly does battle with the forces of oxidation. Leading the charge is perhaps the greatest antioxidant, glutathione. Formed in the liver through the assembly of three amino acids, glutathione assists in the elimination of environmental toxins, protects against oxidation and helps quench inflammation resulting from an overactive immune system.[40] [41] Many autoimmune diseases and brain-based disorders such as ADHD[42] and Alzheimer's[43] are directly associated with low levels of glutathione.

The three amino acids that compose glutathione are: L-glutamine, glycine and cysteine. Generally when glutathione is low, one or more of these amino acids are required, but not all.[44] [45] Certain herbs like Cordyceps found in China, can elevate glutathione levels as well, sometimes dramatically.[46] The body does manufacture certain antioxidants however; whole-food choices still determine how much antioxidant activity is present. This means that a diet replete with different colored vegetables is still at the top of any health list.

NF-KB, METHYLATION AND NITRIC OXIDE

The human body is an amazing amalgam of feedback loops, teeter-totters, and self-governing mechanisms, as discussed throughout *Hope for Health*. Generally, as one process turns on, another process is ready to turn it off (i.e. the inflammation of free radicals is countered by stored antioxidants). When everything is working harmoniously, disease is thwarted and aging is slowed.

The reason inflammation is so damaging is because of its direct effect on cellular mechanisms. Free radicals start a fire of inflammation with unforeseen consequences and collateral damage. Systems designed to regulate cellular function are inevitably caught in the crossfire. Proper nutrition is one way to modulate the cellular damage of aging. Roughly 50 different human genetic diseases arise when the wrong mutant enzymes replace the right B-vitamins, called coenzymes.[47] This disease-promoting cycle is set up when proper levels of B-vitamins are too low and can be remedied when those levels are high.[48] Raising B-vitamin levels prevents the polymorphisms of bad gene replication[49] and many of the diseases of unwanted gene expression.

Damage from inflammation is inevitable, but can be greatly ameliorated with a strong defense of the cellular homeland. Inflammation directly assaults four essential nutrient-based systems critical for proper cellular function. The four systems are the methylation pathway, the nitric oxide system, the eicosanoids and the NF-kB system. The B-vitamins folic acid and B-12 are directly responsible for balancing the methylation pathway. The nitric oxide and NF-kB systems are dependent upon adequate levels of the super antioxidant glutathione, which itself is dependent upon vitamins B6 and B2 and a compound called, sulforaphaneglucosinolate (SGS), found in nature, especially in broccoli plant seeds.[50] Finally, the eicosanoids rely upon sufficient levels and proper ratios of good fats, called essential fatty acids.

The NF-kB System

To recap, anti-aging and longevity means that cells are properly replicating their DNA, while at the same time preventing unwanted gene expression. The process of genetic expression is called transcription and is under the governance a substance called nuclear factor-kappa beta, or the NF-kB system. This regulatory protein is found in almost all animal cell types and is responsive to nearly all cellular stimuli. Too much unwelcome epigenetic influence, such as stress, immune chemicals, free radicals, ultraviolet irradiation, bad cholesterol, and bacterial or viral antigens,[51] [52] speeds up the NF-kB engine and results in the expression of bad genes. This is the friendly way of saying that excess NF-kB activity will lead to cancer, inflammatory and autoimmune diseases, and chronic infections.

The same lifestyle aspects that lengthen telomeres will also slow down NF-kB. The NF-kB system is inhibited by glutathione and a process in the cell called ubiquitination. A supplement known as ubiquinone is one of a group of nutrients responsible for pressing the brake on the NF-kB system, and is easily recognized by its common name, Co-Q-10. A host of popular medications, such as statin drugs for cholesterol, decrease levels of this critical nutrient,[53] which is just one of many reasons to avoid pharmaceuticals whenever possible.

Methylation

Basically, normal metabolic processes – turning one chemical or hormone into another – will always generate waste. Taking out the biochemical trash is the job of a process known as methylation. But it does even more. The importance of methylation has been recognized in the fields of anti-aging and genetics, where researchers have been actively mining this pathway for life-saving nuggets.[54] From a genetic standpoint, methylation protects DNA transcription by stabilizing the NF-kB system.[55]

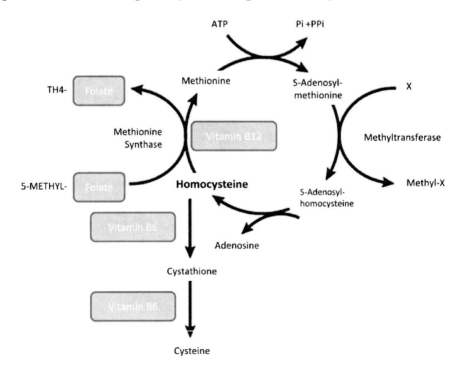

Methyl (CH_3) is a powerful detoxifier of certain chemicals. Both B12 and folic acid have an abundance of it. When needed, these vitamins are able to donate their methyl groups, transforming a potentially harmful substance into something useful or benign. Perhaps the most damaging non-methylated chemical is an amino acid called homocysteine. Research has found that taking high doses of the nutrients B12, B6, and folic acid (folate), reduce homocysteine levels and prevent brain shrinkage in Alzheimer's patients by as much as 50 percent.[56] These nutrients are the principle supporters of the methylation pathway. Because of its direct relationship to heart disease, and vascular damage, homocysteine is discussed further in the chapter, *Panic or Pass Out?*

The Nitric Oxide System

If methylation is faulty from oxidation overload, a third important system related to anti-aging will follow. The chemical nitric oxide (NO) plays a leading role in the control of inflammation by modulating the immune response.[57] It also supports blood flow to the brain, hands, feet[58] and sexual organs,[59] and increases metabolic endurance during exercise.[60] But not all of its impacts are positive. If the damage from free radicals is great enough, glutathione levels will drop and the nitric oxide system will become altered.

NO does its work via three enzymes, called synthases: neuronal NOS (nNOS), endothelial NOS (eNOS) and inducible NOS (iNOS). The first two are very helpful, the last one is not.[61] nNOS for instance, is used to optimize brain function by increasing the growth of new neurons and working specifically at the space between neurons known as the synapse. eNOS aids in the dilation of blood vessels, helps balance blood sugar, and enhances energy utilization by supporting muscle mitochondria. iNOS is the bad guy. Its activity promotes inflammation, arterial plaque build-up and perpetuates free radicals leading to tissue destruction and autoimmune mechanisms.

Research into cellular mechanisms has indicted iNOS and excess nitric oxide as the primary culprits of "unexplained illnesses" such as Chronic

Fatigue Syndrome, Multiple Chemical Sensitivity, Fibromyalgia and Post-Traumatic Stress Disorder.[62] However, their damage is also a major reason for functional illness of all types, which expresses itself long before more complex illness ever shows up. Halting iNOS and balancing nitric oxide is therefore critical for optimizing health. This can be done by increasing glutathione levels, reducing free-radicals, promoting proper methylation and through one other mechanism. The fourth and final system on the anti-aging team has everything to do with the health of the cell itself and is responsible for keeping all cellular occupations functioning properly. These are the eicosanoids.

EICOSANOIDS

Eicosanoids are hormones present in each of the 70 trillion cells of the human body. Rather than endocrine hormones, like estrogen and testosterone, traveling throughout the blood stream, or paracrine hormones communicating between cells, eicosanoids are autocrine hormones. This means they work within the cells themselves, each one having its own special role to play. There are currently around 100 known eicosanoids[63] with names such as prostaglandins, leukotrienes, and thromboxanes. All cellular function (which means all human function) is based on these elusive chemicals. The balance between eicosanoids is what either enhances or degrades health. Most of the top-ten causes of death directly relate to eicosanoid imbalances, including heart disease, hypertension, type 2 diabetes, inflammatory diseases, auto-immune diseases, cancer, depression, and many more.[64] [65] [66] [67]

All eicosanoids are essential, but under certain circumstances, some are much more important and others more harmful. Therefore, if the operating assumption is that most people are not in perfect health, have some degree of emotional stress, and their diet could use some improvement, then the title of "good" and "bad" eicosanoids becomes applicable.

"Good" Eicosanoids	"Bad" Eicosanoids
Inhibit platelet aggregation	Promote platelet aggregation
Vasodilators	Vasoconstrictors
Anti-inflammatory	Pro-inflammatory
Control cellular proliferation	Promote cellular proliferation
Encourage immune function	Suppress immune function

So how is it possible to manipulate eicosanoids naturally for the benefit of improved function? By understanding how the body makes them. All eicosanoids come from oils called essential fatty acids (EFAs). "Essential" means that the body cannot make these oils. They must come from the diet. The irony is that EFAs are useful, or become activated, after oxidization. That's right. The process that damages DNA and creates free radicals, leading to inflammation, is the very same process used to kick-start the production of anti-inflammatory eicosanoids.

It makes good biological sense that oils would contain a key to health and anti-aging. Oil is human soil, or the environment from which health springs forth. The brain is 50 percent fats and oils. All the nerves throughout the nervous system have a coating of fat, called a myelin sheath. Fat makes all hormones, whether within the cell itself or floating around the blood stream. Every cell in the body has as its membrane a double-dose of fat called a bilipid layer.

The cell membrane is Grand Central Station. Without a healthy cell membrane, nutrients do not move in and waste products do not move out of the cell. But this is just for starters. Hormones, nutrients, chemicals of all kinds, and even light waves engage the cell membrane and elicit a response through specific receptor proteins. Cellular biologists believe that there may be more than 100,000 of these proteins, each designed to respond to a precise environmental stimulus.[68] Keeping the plethora of processes moving efficiently requires a healthy cell membrane, and this is dependent upon access to an abundance of essential oils - the same oils required to make good eicosanoids. Harvesting good eicosanoids and weeding out bad ones must be the foundation of any anti-aging program.

Since the early 1980s, researchers have known about eicosanoids and have used oils with mixed results to try to balance their levels for the benefit of health. This is not surprising. The power and success of oils is based upon two important caveats. First, not just any oil will do. Second, the oils used must be ingested in the correct ratios. These ratios can vary from one person to the next, depending on the present state of health. Overall, it is a delicate scale, easily tipped in one direction or another. Overdosing either side, even with good oils, will create problems.

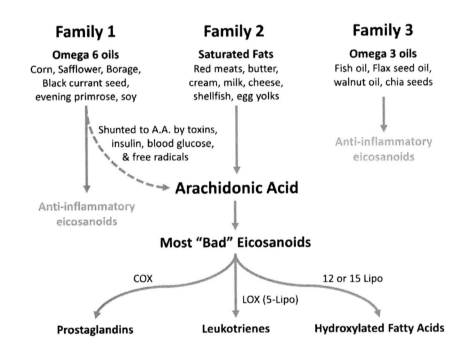

There are three families of oils that can make eicosanoids. Family 1 and Family 3 are where most good eicosanoids come from, while Family 2 produces most bad eicosanoids.

Family 1 is full of omega 6 oils that come from a variety of plants and vegetable-based foods. Family 3 has the omega 3 fats, like fish and flax seed oils. Fish oils have the ability to protect the heart and reduce the incidence of cardiac arrest.[69] [70] They do this by reducing the inflammatory response.[71] [72] However, just taking fish oils is not enough for optimal function. In order for eicosanoids to diminish inflammation, they often need to be present in the correct ratio, balanced against the omega 6 oils of Family 1.[73] [74]

Family 2 are the fats cardiologists want all their patients to avoid, like saturated fats found in red meats, butters, and creams. These fats easily and directly convert into arachidonic acid. While arachidonic acid is critical for brain development in children and has many other important functions throughout life, the eicosanoids from arachidonic acid can make things much worse by increasing pain, constricting blood vessels, and promoting blood clots. This usually occurs when inflammation becomes aggressive. However, there is more to the story. The whole truth of Family 2 fats—and why avoiding them is a Band-Aid approach that may in fact be detrimental—is discussed in the chapter *Fueled or Fatty*.

From arachidonic acid, three main groups of eicosanoids emerge. The first group is the prostaglandins. These are the eicosanoids whose production is shut down by NSAIDS, like acetaminophen and ibuprofen. They do this by not allowing an enzyme to do its job. Enzymes are like workers on an assembly line. As the protein and fat pieces flow down the line, enzymes put them together. Drugs like NSAIDS prevent workers from showing up to work. One enzyme responsible for putting together bad eicosanoids is Cyclooxygenase-1, or COX-1. NSAIDS are COX-1 inhibitors. This may sound like a good idea at first. Who needs enzymes putting together bad eicosanoids anyway? The problem is COX-1 also assembles good eicosanoids, such as the ones that keep the stomach from digesting itself. Too many COX-1 inhibitors will often lead to gastro-intestinal bleeding.

Two other eicosanoid groups also come from arachidonic acid: the leukotrienes and the hydroxylated fatty acids. NSAIDS do nothing to help these last two. The pharmaceutical industry is working on a new class of

LOX enzyme inhibitors to prevent leukotriene formation. Natural LOX inhibitors, such as curcumin, fish oils, and certain antioxidants, all come from a good diet. However, few choose that approach exclusively. If persistent pain is coming from leukotrienes or hydroxylated fatty acids, a common approach in today's fix-me-now society is to go nuclear with steroids.

Steroid drugs, like those prescribed by Rheumatologists, do work to stop pain by shutting off bad eicosanoid production. However, they do more than this. Steroids shut off all eicosanoid function—good and bad. People on steroid drugs often gain weight, become depressed, have trouble sleeping, develop brittle bones, and so on. To reiterate, eicosanoids regulate all human function by controlling cellular function. Shutting the inflammatory and anti-inflammatory eicosanoids down at the same time with steroid drugs has a negative impact on the whole body. This will not, and does not, end well.

Eat Balanced Amounts of Good Oils

The American diet is full of too many omega 6 oils. All the oils in the boxed and bagged goods of the grocery store are omega 6 vegetable oils. This is undesirable for two reasons. First, these oils are all the same types: corn oil and soy bean oil, mostly. It is never a good idea to eat the same things all the time, even if they are good for you. A variety of good foods is best. Second, oils in processed foods have lost any value they once had due to high heat and exposure to oxygen. High heat changes the molecular structure of the oil, making it poisonous in some cases. Oxygen causes free radical damage, turning the oils rancid.

Besides the two reasons just given, omega 6 oils can easily convert into arachidonic acid with a deficiency of omega 3 oils. This tends to happen in the presence of a blood sugar problem, such as insulin resistance. To balance the teeter-totter, physicians have prescribed heavy doses of omega 3 fish oil. This approach works well at first but soon creates other imbalances. Good eicosanoids come from both the omega 6 and omega 3 oils, not just fish oils alone. Generally, the body wants good sources of both omega 6 and omega 3 oils in order to keep inflammatory eicosanoid levels low. Using both families of oils, along with reducing or eliminating bad fats and heated omega 6 oils is the best approach. However, there are other potholes to watch out for.

Rolling Toward Inflammation

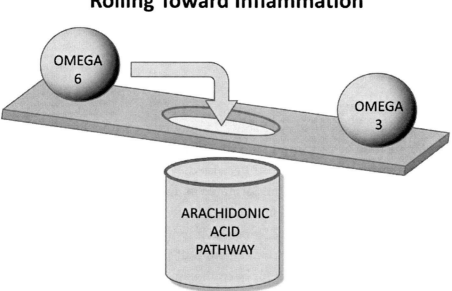

Avoid Bad Fats

Not all fats are equal. Man-made synthetic and processed fats (trans fats) greatly disrupt eicosanoid balance, increase inflammation, and interfere with cholesterol breakdown. As such, people should avoid eating them. The process of partial hydrogenation changes the shapes of natural fats and oils so they interfere with, rather than promote, normal fat metabolism. A study published in the New England Journal of Medicine estimates that simply eliminating trans fats from the U.S. food supply could prevent between 6 and 19 percent of heart attacks and related deaths, or more than 200,000 deaths each year.[75]

These processed fats are in nearly everything people buy in the grocery store, from salad dressings to candy bars and from chips to breads.

Partially hydrogenated fats and oils block the normal conversion of cholesterol in the liver, causing an elevation of cholesterol in the blood. Margarine, which is often touted for its lack of cholesterol, contains partially hydrogenated fats. One of the biggest cases of misinformation in recent history is the suggestion that eating margarine instead of butter will reduce cholesterol. It is true that butter contains cholesterol and that margarine does not. But, butter also contains high levels of normal fat mobilizing nutrients. It is a whole food designed to take care of its own fats if eaten in moderation. Margarine can actually increase cholesterol levels and heart attacks.[76]

Watch Out for Sugar

Some people can eat plenty of Family 2 saturated fat without any evidence of inflammation or its scariest outcome, heart disease. How is this counter-intuitive trend possible? Because they don't over-ingest sugars and have normal blood insulin. Saturated fat by itself is neutral or can be anti-inflammatory but not when combined with sugars.[77] [78] Americans love sweets and grease. In the Standard American Diet, saturated fat is rarely unaccompanied by copious amounts of sugar. With each dessert, Americans increase their risk for heart disease,[79] [80] eating roughly 150 pounds of refined sweeteners each year.[81] Too much sugar leads to spikes in the sugar-regulating hormone insulin. This hormone has the strongest influence over the eicosanoids. Too much insulin as a result of too much sugar is a trigger for functional illness. The majority of people, as discussed in the chapter *Hypoglycemia or Histamine,* have a functional blood sugar problem that is pushing them toward life-altering disease.

Sugars with Family 2 fats are bad enough, but to add fuel to the inflammatory fire, simply change Family 2 fats to the bad trans fats. Since 1920, the percentage of dietary vegetable oils in the form of margarine, shortening, and refined oils increased nearly 400 percent while the consumption of sugar and processed foods increased about 60 percent.[82] Studies from around the world have consistently demonstrated that in populations where the diet was high in sugar, processed flours, and heated vegetable oils, deaths from all manner of disease, including heart disease, are much higher.[83] [84] [85] [86] [87]

A Final Piece

In the body, everything is about balance between systems: not too hot, not too cold. Avoiding bad oils and consuming good oils is a great start and will pay dividends. However, maximum effect from oils, the kind of effect that helps cure arthritis, eczema, and colitis, results when people consume both omega 3 and omega 6 oils at the same time *in their correct ratios.*

Diagnostic blood tests can determine the levels of EFAs in the body. However, the levels of these oils are different within different types of body tissues. This means that blood tests, as helpful as they may be, still leave many critical questioned unanswered.

Which type of omega 3 oil is best: flax seed oil, cod liver oil, or a combined fish oil product? Which type of omega 6 oil is best: black currant seed oil or borage oil? Or perhaps evening primrose oil, wheat germ oil, or some combination of the above? And of course, how much of each? Two fish oil to one borage, or the other way around? Finally, will the patient actually be able to digest all these oils and use them efficiently in the body? The answers to these questions will lay a foundation for health and anti-aging.

Conclusion

Summarizing what has been learned so far: The things that make us sick are the same things that accelerate aging. The reason this is so is because all diseases and functional imbalances originate from dysfunction in the cells. When cells are stressed, replication increases and total cellular lifespan decreases. Slowing biological aging begins with a strong defense of DNA against inflammatory assault. The main threats come from oxidation-generated free radicals, poor cellular methylation, an overactive NF-kB system, a skewed nitric oxide system and inadequate levels of good eicosanoids. To prevent aging the fundamental processes of cellular replication and transcription must be guarded.

- Telomeres must be kept as long as possible with proper health and lifestyle habits.
- The inflammation from free radicals must be minimized with antioxidants.
- The methylation and nitric oxide pathways must be properly maintained.
- The brakes of the NF-kB system must be engaged with co-Q-10 and glutathione.
- The cell membrane must be kept pliable and elastic and inflammatory eicosanoids must be reduced with the proper ratio of essential fatty acids.

Each of the dangers and their foundational counter steps are pictured in the figure below.

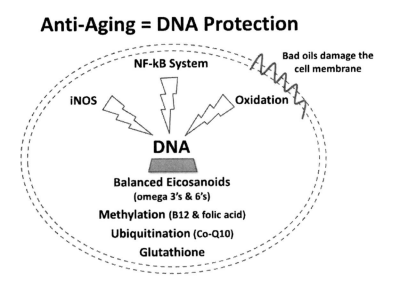

Anti-Aging = DNA Protection

Figure 2: Protecting DNA

At this point some may conclude that anti-aging is just a bit too complicated. Telomeres? Methylation? Oxidation? Eicosanoids? Where does one begin? The body is, in one way, simple. It will thrive when it gets what it needs and avoids what it doesn't. But it is in no way simplistic. What exactly does it need and what should it avoid? The answer is often different for different people, but there is an answer. The wonderful news is that a fascinating whole-person healing approach can determine the things required to restore health.

It is time to discover this new world, one that modern diagnostic equipment can in some cases confirm but cannot replicate; a world that is explained through neurology, neurochemistry, bioenergetics, epigenetics, and in some cases, quantum mechanics. A world that, once understood, will advance health by changing the way people eat, think, and live. It is time to discover Functional Bio-Analysis.

FUNCTIONAL BIO-ANALYSIS – WHAT, HOW, WHY?

WHAT IS IT?

This chapter of *Hope for Health* details how Functional Bio-Analysis is even possible. It may be a bit complex, but this is necessary for academic reasons and to satisfy the natural questions generated by such a topic. However, some of you may want to start by flipping through the *Table of Contents* or the *Index* to find the greatest areas of concern in your own life. Turn to those pages and see how FBA works through the natural metabolic pathways to find the cause and the cure. Then, return to *Functional Bio-Analysis – What? How? Why?* for detailed explanations of how it is all possible.

Since the 1960s, alternative medicine, in its various forms, has advanced in U.S. culture. During this time, the interest in all things "natural" led to an explosion of alternative healing techniques, many of which had no scientific foundation. These techniques failed to withstand speculation, evaluation and attack, proving to be little more than fads or trends. In the competitive world of health care, those alternative techniques that have endured have done so by their own merits. The fact they are still here at present, despite conspiratorial attacks to eliminate some of them,[88] demonstrates they have received the stamp of approval from the public at large and now no longer carry the somewhat derogatory title of "alternative" but are instead complementary.

Applied Kinesiology (AK) is one technique that has survived. AK, despite past and present efforts to discredit its efficacy, has endured due to its success in areas where traditional medicine has failed and continues to fail. At its core, AK was the first technique to incorporate the manual muscle test, or MMT,[89] as one of its primary methods of evaluation, believing *practitioners can use the muscles of the body as an analytical tool to evaluate human function.*[90]

With this realization, vast implications were foreseen and not surprisingly, many offshoots were conceived. Emerging under the "kinesiology" banner, techniques such as Clinical Kinesiology, Quantum Kinesiology, Nutrition Response Testing and Muscle Response Testing[91] were born. Competition between these groups led to new discoveries, refinements and innovations, making already good procedures more efficient and effective. The worlds of biochemistry, neurology and nutritional research kept pace as well, providing the scientific foundation upon which the regular breakthroughs could rest. Pioneers in AK such as Dr. Walter Schmitt,[92] Dr. Chris Astil-Smith,[93] and Dr. Michael Lebowitz[94] developed entire protocols and techniques to address the biochemistry and nutritional needs of the body. Their work, and that of many others, is the foundation upon which FBA now stands.

Functional Bio-Analysis (FBA) is a science-based complementary medicine technique, helping knowledgeable practitioners navigate the neurological and energetic pathways present in all people. The primary goal of FBA is to tap into the body's own natural monitoring system in order to evaluate the functions within. FBA, like AK, is done with precise manual muscle testing.

With FBA, practitioners can follow ordered steps to find the nutrients the body needs most. This approach produces a hormetic effect. Hormesis has Greek origins and means, "to set in motion, impel, or urge on." A hormetic nutrient may be a single vitamin, herb or other agent that positively impacts multiple systems simultaneously.

One of the first things an FBA practitioner will do is find the primary energetic points (PEPs). These points are well known and have been used for thousands of years in classical acupuncture. With FBA, it is possible to identify the PEPs with the highest priority and then all the remaining PEPs in their order of importance. Through this hierarchy, health professionals can address the primary things first, saving time and resources often wasted on less significant issues.

Along the body's structured pathway, there are many other fascinating and pertinent tests an experienced practitioner can add as he or she deems necessary according to the symptoms and metabolic needs of the patient. For instance, the three primary colors of the visual spectrum (green, red and violet) relate to specific genetic tendencies. Each color is associated with a major organ weakness and food intolerance as well as with other health-disrupting tendencies. Just knowing these pieces of information would help millions of people manage and maintain their health. (For more information, see the chapter, *What Color Are You?*). There are also eight eye positions, which reveal whether major minerals such as calcium, magnesium, iron and zinc are out of balance; and numerous soft-tissue tests that make known the integrity of the skin, hair and joints.

The success of FBA practitioners is dependent upon their knowledge of physiologic pathways, their ability to use the craft of manual muscle testing and their knowledge of standard and special diagnostic tests. In fact, FBA is the perfect bridge between the worlds of functional and energetic medicine. Functional medicine doctors analyze standard diagnostic tests, such as blood work, and then recommend natural remedies. Energetic medicine doctors utilize the body itself as a diagnostic tool: FBA practitioners do both.

FOUR KEY PRINCIPLES

FBA operates on four key principles. **First**, when a functional imbalance or even a disease is present, it indicates the brain/body has recognized and pinpointed the problem, but for a variety of reasons, lacks the means to restore its own balance, or homeostasis. When this occurs, it does the next best thing—it reveals the areas in need via well recognized energetic points located on acupuncture meridians. The FBA practitioner needs only to follow the manifested energetic road map as revealed through the PEPs in order to locate the most significant imbalances.

Second, there is a hierarchy. In other words, the body knows what it needs fixed first and the order thereafter. This is critical. Most techniques will start at the patient's complaint. However, most complaints are downstream problems. Locating the headwaters and addressing the issues found at the source is the approach that produces "miracles."

Third, fixing the ordered steps along the way requires hormetic nutrients. These are the foundational nutrients that affect vast numbers of metabolic functions. Hormetic nutrients do the heavy lifting and include specific forms of nutrients such as calcium, magnesium, B6, folic acid and many others. Utilizing hormetic nutrients exclusively will make recovery faster and more permanent and prevent Shopping Bag Syndrome (SBS), the rapidly growing phenomenon of using a shopping-bag's worth of daily supplements as part of one's health routine.

Fourth, manual muscle testing is currently the only method of human analysis available to navigate the body's energetic healing map according to its revealed priority. However, proper manual muscle testing is essential to acquire accurate data and avoid false findings—an all too common occurrence.

MANUAL MUSCLE TESTING (MMT) - HOW IS IT POSSIBLE?

Considering the four principles above, the one that generates the most confusion and perhaps ire is manual muscle testing. The theory behind MMT is fully compatible with the classical understanding of neurology, physiology and electromagnetic principles.[95] There are no concepts based on mysterious forces or that lack a scientific rationale. **MMT is simply a change in the tone of a muscle from strong (facilitated) to weak (inhibited), or from weak to strong, in the presence of a given stimulus.**

Many of the theories explaining how muscle testing works, its validity and its meaning to the rest of the body, have sprung from Applied Kinesiology. Researchers and practitioners have studied these theories for decades.[96] In classical AK teaching, all muscles have a relationship with an organ, as indicated in the following chart.

Muscle	Related Organ
Pectoralis Major Sternal	Liver
Middle Deltoid	Lungs
Quadriceps	Small Intestine
Hamstrings	Large Intestine

Table 1: Examples of Muscle/Organ Relationships

The connections between the muscles and the organs above are just a small piece of the phenomenon called *Bio-unity*. This simply means that every part connects to every other part, and every system connects to every other system. Because of this inter-connected relationship, a change or modification in any one part will have a corresponding effect on every other part. If the theory of Bio-unity holds true, a practitioner should be able to find that any major imbalance, be it a nutritional deficiency, emotional disturbance, inflammatory response or anything else, will be manifested in the body through various systems. For instance, if a person has an inflammatory condition, a doctor can perform a blood test to check for certain inflammatory chemicals, such as C-reactive protein and homocysteine. These are the chemical signs, but are there neurological, energetic, neuromuscular and even emotional signs of inflammation? The answer is yes. This reality is consistent for any imbalance within the body.

A good illustration is the state of depression. The neuromuscular sign with depression is a slumped posture, the chemical sign is low serotonin, the energetic sign is a disrupted flow through the bladder meridian, the neurological sign has to do with specific disruptions in right- and left-brain function and the emotional sign is the depression itself. In other words, all the systems of the body have a road map the practitioner may follow in order to arrive at the patient's most pressing needs. Some roads are easier to traverse than others. FBA is based on the concepts of Bio-unity and utilizes MMT to tap into these systems in an orderly, repeatable and reproducible fashion.

With Bio-unity, evaluating groups of muscles and finding weaknesses where strength should be present could provide significant insight into the general function of the body. For instance, a strong chest muscle called the pectoralis major sternal, or PMS, is related to the liver.[97] If something compromises liver function in some way, it is likely the function of the PMS muscle will also be less than optimal and likely will not test strong.

For the purposes of this book, MMT moves a step further. Practitioners can use FBA to not only analyze the muscles themselves but also every substance that influences physiologic function such as hormones, neurotransmitters, environmental chemicals and even foods. It is possible for the body to evaluate these minute substances, because it is able to detect and react to whatever stimulus is present through an intricate and fascinating process outside of the five senses.

Most people understand the human body detects stimuli through taste, touch, smell, sound and sight. What they may not understand is the plethora of subtle yet meaningful changes taking place when each of these senses is stirred, or the even more powerful detection system that governs all the body does and is capable of doing. **This detection system goes beyond the five senses to a sixth sense, an electromagnetic sense that can detect a substance via its natural and ever-present electrical emanations.**

In reality, the human body is so sensitive there need not be a substance at all. Just a thought or an emotion could be enough to generate a change in muscle response. But before going too far with a discussion on these intriguing phenomena, one should comprehend the foundation for the technique.

The skeptic doubts the possibility a small stimulus such as a smell, taste or thought could be a profound enough trigger in the nervous system to alter the tone of a strong muscle, making it temporarily weak. And as for a substance merely in contact with the body doing the same thing, clearly the skeptic would find this idea is not believable. The criticism seems reasonable on its face, because it appears to fit everyday experience. No one, they would argue, has suddenly fallen to the floor after smelling peanuts, petting a cat or breathing in pollen. How then could someone say that these same things could make the muscle of an allergic person shut off when they are simply exposed to them? And yet, this is exactly what happens every day in offices of muscle testing practitioners across the country and the world.

So, how is this possible? Is it the trickery of the practitioner as he shamelessly manipulates the unsuspecting patient with sleight of hand and mesmeristic maneuvers? Or, are there very real and significant phenomena taking place that are poorly understood and yet profound concerning the function of the human body and even the future potential of medicine?

THE BODY REACTS TO EVERYTHING

Much of the body's adaptation to the environment is performed automatically through reflexes. Reflexes are one form of biofeedback. The biofeedback measured with MMT is similar to reflex responses experienced every moment through the five senses. The scientific world[98] well understands reflexive responses and groups them into several categories.[99] Stretch reflexes, or deep tendon reflexes, are the kind doctors test when tapping the end of the knee with a rubber hammer.[100] Superficial reflexes alert the body to the slightest changes in sensation. Visceral, or autonomic, reflexes help the body to regulate changes in light or blood pressure. So-called primitive reflexes help to keep people from falling and help babies to root and suck.[101] In other words, **if the body needs it, there is a reflex to help achieve it; if the body can sense it, there is a reflex to help protect against it.**

Examples of reflexes from the five senses are familiar, since they fit everyday experience. Everyone has been hungry, smelled a pleasant food and experienced salivation and the stomach rumblings that followed. An unpleasant smell or taste, on the other hand, elicits a strong and immediate negative reflexive reaction: squinting of the face and jerking back the head as if to pull away. These are the involuntary responses common with exposure to pleasant and unpleasant stimuli.[102] An experience—even when recalled through memory alone—creates an instant physiological and emotional change. If the memory is enjoyable, the response may be a smile, laugh or "warm feeling." If the memory is upsetting, recognizable emotional and physical signs will manifest.

If an emotional stimulus is long lasting, profound signs may be present. For example, depression generates a slumped posture with shoulders rolled forward, head tilted down and torso bent slightly forward;[103] whereas, the opposite is present in a proud or confident person who, in a military fashion, stands straight and tall with his shoulders rolled back. These responses demonstrate generally that **the body reacts through its muscles to stimuli.** With this basic tenet established, it is now safe to move into more precise illustrations.

To prevent injury, the body has a sophisticated neurological warning system to protect itself from mechanical injury, i.e. strains, sprains and soft tissue tears. Located in the musculotendinous junction, the place where the muscle stops and the tendon starts, are specialized cells called golgi tendon organs (GTOs). They are kill switches, and it is their job to turn off a contracting muscle if it pulls too hard and/or to protect the muscle no matter how intense the contraction. If GTOs weren't there, tendons would rip from bones during extreme exertion, or the muscle could continue to contract at the onset of injury, when ceasing to contract would be more beneficial.[104] So when injury is imminent, the GTOs signal the brain, which turns off the contracting muscle through a process called the autogenic inhibition reflex.[105] Likewise there are kill switches in the middle, or belly, of all muscles called spindle cells. Their job is to prevent overstretching. This is called the stretch reflex.[106] If a muscle is in the process of being overstretched, the muscle spindles signal the brain, which shuts off all the opposing muscles creating the stretch. These examples show something very important with regard to the validity of manual muscle testing: **There are neurologically understood ways in which the body voluntarily turns off its own muscles in response to stimuli, especially those stimuli it deems potentially harmful.**

So far, the examples have shown the body responds through its muscles to stimuli via built-in reflexes and confirmed the body does so immediately and in very different ways depending on the nature of the stimulus, good or bad, healthy or harmful. But what about the big question? What about energetic stimuli—those not detected by the five senses? Is the human body sensitive enough to perceive and protect itself from them the same way it can to mechanical stimulation? The answer to this question rests in three things: First, understanding the capabilities of the nervous system; second, in the microscopic properties of all substances; and third, in the complexities of cellular systems that are poorly understood but profoundly significant.

THE BODY EVALUATES EVERYTHING

To protect itself against unwanted or harmful changes, the human body must monitor and react to its environment at every instant. With each breath, bite or thought, chemical changes occur at the cellular level. Scientists are now broadening their diagnostic scope by using trained dogs to detect certain cancers[107] based on evidence showing the disease has its own smell, different from the normal tissue. Researchers in this field of study are using dogs to detect the presence of lung,[108,109] ovarian[110] and colorectal cancers.[111] This ground-breaking form of analysis reveals that even the smallest changes at the cellular level are measurable if given the right "nose." Diagnostic methods that can find pathologies without being invasive would be a blessing to patients and their wallets. But it gets even more amazing.

Most of the "thinking" done by the body is the unconscious. Even while awake, the unconscious mind monitors 95 percent or more of the total stimulation the body experiences. When the eyes are focused on an object a few feet away, most of what is present in the peripheral vision is unnoticed—it is not processed consciously. It is easy enough to bring the unconscious to the conscious. The simple wave of a hand in the periphery or the passing of a moving object could be enough visual input to cause the mind to shift focus, resulting in a quick head turn to see this new thing. In other words, the whole world is being monitored and evaluated at every instant, but only a small portion actually generates a response. This seems basic enough; however, the true complexity of this process begins to come to light when attempting to estimate just how many processes the body evaluates each second.

Temperature, pressure, light, sound, smells, thoughts, impressions, decisions and voluntary movements are just some of the categories of information under scrutiny within the body. Unconsciously, it evaluates at any living moment every one of the 100 trillion[112] cells and their metabolic activity. Every hormone, every step in energy production, digestion, blood sugar management, immune system regulation, thyroid activity, energy creation, pain management, emotional balance and more are under continuous assessment and modification. This is truly fantastic, but true all the same.

Inside a cell there are thousands of protein-based enzymes at work continuously.[113] A conservative approximation for the number of processes underway each second would be tens of thousands. To get an idea of the total number of processes the body must monitor we would need to take this number and multiply it by the total number of cells. The result is in the neighborhood of 10^{16} reactions per second. Putting this number in perspective, there are an estimated 10^{22} atoms in the human body and the same number of stars in the universe. This is an incomprehensible and seemingly limitless amount of information under the body's governorship.

Accounting for all of this, scientists, for close to a century now, have believed and taught that all the reactions within a cell and then throughout the rest of the body happened as chemicals accidentally contacted each other in the ambiguous cellular open spaces. When this occurred, the theory claimed electrons jumped their orbits, creating new molecules. The whole thing supposedly happened in a *random* but orderly fashion. Just the numerical facts already presented should lead one to question whether a haphazard, "bump-and-switch" physiology is a sufficient explanation for the level of complexity and detail now known to exist. It is not.

The accepted random-chemical explanation for how physiological processes are directed in the human body is wholly insufficient simply because no understood chemical reactions happen fast enough via random contact to sustain life at its current pace and overall rate of response. If accidental chemical reactions were the only explanation for human physiology, the current speed of life would be impossible. Prudence now suggests another explanation: **A whole-body system must exist that is able to assimilate the deluge of ever-present internal and external stimuli and then generate a response to this surge instantaneously.**

EVERYTHING IS ELECTROMAGNETIC

Food passed under the nose of a blindfolded man is easily identified by its unique smell. A sample of food placed in the mouth could just as easily be recognized by its unique taste. The point is, an apple never tastes like an orange, and chocolate doesn't taste like a pretzel. Everything has its own unique characteristics because of its constituent components – what it is made of. The five senses are the best known means of classifying substances based on their distinctive characteristics, but there is an even more mysterious method of identification.

Any substance a person can call a solid is made up of atoms, which are then made up of smaller substances called protons, neutrons and electrons. The electrons can travel at close to the speed of light[114] and do so in their orbit around the protons and neutrons located near the center, or nucleus of an atom. Amazingly, the space between the electrons and the nucleus is much greater than the charged particles themselves, by a factor of ten million to one.[115] It is in this area the electrons do their microscopic dance. To get an idea of how this dance is choreographed, if a human dancer, representing an electron, was shrunk to about two feet tall, her dance floor would be the size of the earth. And, she would dance around the entire land surface seven times every second.

This illustration reveals something very important with regards to the physical world. Most of what is considered solid is not really solid at all, but is actually more empty space than material, a whole lot more. Knowing these mathematical facts, it is a wonder the chair can hold the sitter; the cup can hold the coffee; and when the mailman knocks at the door, his hand doesn't pass right on through! It is the powerful electrical and magnetic forces that allow subatomic particles to move certain distances, but no further, giving them the relative-reality of being solid.

If that were not mind-expanding enough, in terms of quantum mechanics, everything in the universe is energy, and energy is either a force or a transport medium for information. Through sight and sound, frequencies are the source of most communication in life. Right now, the eyes detect the words on this page via reflected light. Light, via the electromagnetic spectrum, is the source of most frequencies whether the waves are radio, microwave, infrared, visible, ultraviolet, X-ray or gamma. Nearly all of the electronic communication that takes place on the earth is via radio or television waves.[116] Other frequencies also carry information. Sound waves result from vibrations generated through a speaker or when objects collide or just pass by each other, as is the case with air moving along the vocal chords. The idea that frequencies transmit information is a critical concept for the validation of muscle testing with FBA for one very important reason: *all* substances generate and emit frequencies as part of an electromagnetic field.

Producing an electromagnetic field requires two things: an electric charge and motion.[117] This is precisely the constitution of all matter - rapidly moving, negatively charged electrons spinning around positively charged protons and uncharged neutrons. As it turns out, electromagnetic fields are not some strange phenomenon, but are instead one of the foundational principles of all substances. So much so, electromagnetic fields are considered one of the four fundamental forces of nature (the others being gravity, the weak nuclear interaction and the strong nuclear interaction).

The electromagnetic field is unique to a substance and is therefore as much of an identifying marker as is its taste or smell. In other words, **the electromagnetic field of a substance is its energetic fingerprint.** Additionally, since electromagnetic fields create frequencies, and frequencies are a principal means of carrying information, then all substances, without interruption, endlessly announce their identity via their unique electromagnetic fields.

The human body behaves according to the laws of nature. And the laws of nature are undergirded by an electromagnetic reality. Therefore, it should be no surprise that the body operates within and as part of an electromagnetic platform. Thankfully, it appears science is now able to demonstrate what has always been present. Advanced technologies have been designed to study the outer universe of space for scientific purposes and the inner universe of the human body for medical purposes.

All matter will either absorb energy or radiate it back through a process called nuclear magnetic resonance (NMR).[118] The resonance of a material, just like its electromagnetic field, is specific to that substance. Many scientific techniques make use of NMR to study molecular physics, crystals and non-crystalline materials through NMR spectroscopy.[119] By directing energy such as specific radio frequencies at the human body or a blood sample and then measuring the resonance that bounces back, scientists have been able to develop technologies which can identify different types of tissues and even the individual components of human blood. Magnetic resonance imaging, or MRI, is a well-known example. Physicians have used it for decades to peer into the human body and "see" the bones and soft tissues.

The NMR LipoProfile,[120] another sophisticated test using the principle of natural resonance, helps determine whether a patient may be at risk for a heart attack by evaluating the 15 specific kinds of lipoprotein subclasses.[121] [122] These technologies confirm that all substances have a measurable, invisible, energetic specificity, or fingerprint, based upon their unique components; and that these energies are to some degree measurable. But there is much more.

All of civilized society is controlled, arranged and micromanaged by an electromagnetic world which cannot be seen and is poorly understood by its inhabitants. Right now in any urban area there are around 100 million information-packed frequencies passing by and through each resident. These are called electromagnetic frequencies or EMFs. Mobile phones, wireless Internet, satellite signals and radio and television transmissions permeate the space all around, passing through us mostly unnoticed. What is amazing and pertinent to this discussion is that **each of these forms of communication is electromagnetic and invisible and carries mega quantities of information instantaneously over vast distances and through solids; and they do it all with a relatively small power source.** [123]

A mobile signal for instance, can reach a cell tower several miles away. The world that only 50 years ago needed an office building to house the first computer, which could barely add and subtract, takes all these facts for granted. The irony of technology is, that even with its overwhelming complexity, the more people take it for granted, the less they understand it. The same could be said for the human body.

The toys of everyday life like computers, cell phones and MP3 Players, with all of their amazing capabilities, look merely like a pile of wooden blocks when compared to the complexity of living things. At any given moment, a single human cell is operating at a greater rate of complexity than all of New York City, or if the DNA is considered, perhaps more than the entire world.[124] The body has more than 100 trillion such cells[125] all working in harmony for the good of the whole to maintain homeostasis.

Extensive discussion has taken place over whether EMFs are harmful to both animals and humans. Biologists have documented that biological organisms have a high-sensitivity to tiny electrical stimuli. Animals of all sizes use energetic cues to orient themselves geographically during migrations; to locate prey, predators and mates; and to anticipate all sorts of meteorological and geological phenomena such as strong storms, hurricanes, seasonal changes and even earthquakes.[126] [127] [128] Therefore many biologists worry the ever-increasing levels of EMFs will create confusion for classes of animals that rely on specific energetic stimuli to survive. Others worry that these same EMF levels are disrupting human physiology.

High EMF levels have been a health discussion in this country and around the world for many years. Some researchers and authors believe prolonged EMF exposure can contribute to a range of health issues[129] including sleep disorders, depression, ADD, autism, fatigue, bedwetting, nervous disorders and diseases such as leukemia[130] and cancer.[131]

In rebuttal, many scientists consistently state that EMFs are not harmful unless they are able to heat and radiate tissues, causing ionization. They also believe that weak signals, those much less intense than what occurs normally inside tissues, should have no biological effect.[132] Researchers based this logical belief on the reasoning that low levels of stimulation produce small responses and higher levels of stimulation produce higher responses. Surprisingly, this seemingly logical conclusion turns out to be false. **Living systems tend to defy logic. A high percentage of the time weak stimuli produce the largest response, while strong stimuli produce little to no response at all.**[133]

Scientists at the Neuroscience Research Institute examined the evidence and concluded the following information:

A striking range of biological interactions has been described in experiments where control procedures appear to have been adequately considered...the existence of biological effects of very weak electromagnetic fields suggests an extraordinarily efficient mechanism for detecting these fields and discriminating them from much higher levels of noise. The underlying mechanisms must necessarily involve ever increasing numbers of elements in the sensing system, ordered in particular ways to form a cooperative organization and manifesting similar forms and levels of energy over long distances.[134]

These discoveries have led to significant research in the realm of electromagnetic fields and have provided the scientific foundation for the practice of muscle testing and many other forms of energy work. Scientists now understand tissues and cells are non-linear, cooperative, coherent and capable of evaluating and responding to very weak stimuli in a weighty manner.[135] These revelations have in essence proven what alternative medicine practitioners preach and have known for decades. Namely, that the body is able to detect small electromagnetic stimuli and respond to it immediately. One more question remains: exactly how does the body detect electromagnetic fields?

THE LIVING MATRIX

In recent years, seasonal affective disorder (SAD) has gained publicity.[136] SAD is a condition characterized by depression and lack of motivation in individuals who have gone long periods of time without adequate amounts of sunlight. This occurs most often in people who live in northern regions and experience daylight lasting less than 10 hours.[137] When stimulated by sunlight, or even forms of artificial light, a host of functions ensue, including biorhythm regulation,[138] calcium mobilization[139] and pineal gland regulation.[140]

From a health perspective, the consequences of low sunlight levels can be severe and mostly result from a deficiency in vitamin D.[141] The sun also plays a major role in helping the internal body clock, which aids in the release and use of important hormones such as melatonin and serotonin, which are sleep and mood-supporting hormones, respectively. Though the eyes play a major role, the benefits of the sun are not realized with them exclusively. A blind person will suffer the effects of dark winter days just as much as someone who can see.

Studies with light to improve the body clock have demonstrated that photoreceptors, as they are called, are located throughout the entire surface area of the skin.[142] **Remember, visible light is electromagnetic. Therefore, the presence of photoreceptors demonstrates the body does in fact detect, respond to and depend upon electromagnetic energy, with visible light being just one of many such forms.**

All cells have as protection a fatty membrane made up of pairs of phospholipids, which are electrically polarized and arranged in an orderly fashion. This array of similarly polarized structures makes them a potential sensing apparatus, much like a row of radio telescopes that enable astrophysicists to detect extremely weak electromagnetic signals from nebulae thousands of millions of light years away.[143] Many of the body's tissues are arranged in like manner. Collagen in connective tissues, myelin around nerves, contractile tissues in muscles, cilium around hair cells, dendrites in the brain, the rods and cone of the eye, the osteon in bone and sensory endings in retina are just some examples.[144] In fact, every fleck of the human body contains multiple numbers of varying arrays, each with the ability to evaluate electromagnetic stimuli.

Considering the number of arrangements within cellular structures and their potential to interact with electromagnetic stimuli, it seems the body was designed to monitor and respond to its environment not only via the five senses but even more intimately by an omnipresent electromagnetic detection system; what has been called the sixth sense of biology.[145] But there is more. Not only can the body detect and react to the outside world through an electromagnetic network, but it monitors and controls its inner workings through another system just as fascinating.

Early electron microscopy reported that cells appeared to have a large amount of empty space. It was here that enzymes dissolved amino acids and sugars and the known processes of metabolism took place. For decades physiologists have based their research on this premise—a premise, as it turns out, that was entirely simplistic. As electron microscopes improved, a closer look inside the cell demonstrated the empty space had no empty space. Instead it was filled with filaments, tubes, fibers and trabeculaee—collectively called the cytoplasmic matrix, or cytoskeleton.[146]

This inner cytoskeleton contained and protected the enzymes necessary for chemical processes. What's more, the cytoskeleton is not just isolated within the cell itself but is connected to the outside of the cell via linking molecules called *integrins*, which pass through the cell membrane and link to an even greater, more diverse network. **In other words, every cell in the body is connected to every other cell via a living matrix.**

The living matrix is a continuous and dynamic 'supramolecular' webwork, extending into every nook and cranny of the body: a nuclear matrix within a cellular matrix within a connective tissue matrix. In essence, when you touch a human body, you are touching a continuously interconnected system, composed of virtually all of the molecules in the body linked together in an intricate webwork. The living matrix has no fundamental unit or central aspect, no part that is primary or most basic. The properties of the whole net depend upon the integrated activities of all the components. Effects on one part of the system can and do spread to others.

James Oschman, Energy Medicine, The Scientific Basis

These facts about human design and function are a legitimate foundation for the practice of muscle testing and even many forms of energy work. The traditional medical world itself has for decades now, employed electrical and ultrasound based therapies to increase wound healing[147] and reduce pain.[148] Likewise, researchers have discovered that using technology to balance human biofields by reducing potentially harmful EMFs has led to enhanced performance in athletes and anxiety reduction in those under stress.[149]

Given that the world is full of electromagnetic transmissions both natural and man-made; that the character of EMFs allows them to pass through solids, carry incalculable amounts of data and act as the ordinary manifestation of all materials; that with changes in chemistry or physical structure, there will be changes in electrical activity; that the body is able to detect and react to these electromagnetic fingerprints, perhaps even more so than with the other five senses, and does so via an electromagnetic whole-body matrix; that the reactions are often large and significant even though the stimulation may be minute…believing that a substance placed on or near the body might cause a reflex change in the tone of a muscle, may not be such a big leap after all.

WHY FUNCTIONAL BIO-ANALYSIS?

Based on the establishment of a feasible theory for manual muscle testing, another question remains: Why bother with it? Why go to the trouble to train practitioners in its use? Why, with the ever-increasing technology to study human function, is it necessary to have a hands-on method of human assessment?

Reason #1: Functional vs. Pharmaceutical

Traditional allopathic medicine, the kind people have become accustomed to in the United States, is the most technologically advanced form of medicine in the world. It has achieved a strong foothold for a number of reasons. First of all, medicine can and has done a great deal of good, including eliminating and holding at bay many diseases. This is recognized worldwide. When it becomes a matter of life and death, people will leave their home country and travel to the United States to receive the best modern medicine can offer. In addition, today's medicine is easy for the patient. The ideas of taking a pill to eliminate symptoms and of lying asleep on a table and then waking up better are very appealing. There is little or no effort involved.

Furthermore, medicine is exciting, even glamorous. Just think, any day now there may be a medical breakthrough or cure for one of the world's most heinous diseases. Imagine all the scientists in all the major universities around the world peering through their microscopes, testing new compounds and making new discoveries. No wonder society so reveres medical doctors. Consider all the Hollywood celebrities raising money to find a cure for this or that disease. Participation in the funding of scientific research allows the public to be part of the movement to find a cure. These efforts are gratifying and in many cases prove to be fruitful.

Next, insurance pays for traditional medicine. Despite what has been proclaimed, most people have some form of insurance coverage through work, a spouse, Medicare or Medicaid. Access to insurance is often a double edged sword. Having the bills paid for a catastrophic illness or injury is certainly a good thing. However, expecting coverage for even the most minor issues and receiving that coverage at little or no cost, has resulted in a population less proactive with their health. Promoting a symptom-minded, rather than prevention-minded perspective has been a good way to keep people dependent on traditional medical care. Unfortunately, this same approach guarantees a culture ignorant of basic human function and maintenance, which in the long-term will mean more disease with even greater costs.

Finally, there are many individuals, including those who practice complimentary medicine, who have benefited from surgical "miracles." When appropriately practiced, medicine can accomplish great things like saving a mother and child from complications during pregnancy. FBA practitioners are in no way interested in replacing medicine. Instead, they hope to improve and enhance what is already in place.

One way to begin building the symbiotic relationship is by defining the scope of both traditional and complementary medicine. Understanding the capacity of each would be a great help for patients when considering which type of doctor to see for their given ailment. The definitions could establish a clear boundary, demarcating the strengths and weaknesses of each approach. For traditional medicine, many would argue, a weakness would include the area of functional illness.

Currently in our society there is an epidemic of functional imbalances that, if left untreated, will become recognizable diseases. Diabetes, heart disease, stroke and cancer, which account for most of the natural causes of death,[150] all had their start as functional problems that were potentially 100 percent preventable.

It is common for people to describe significant symptoms to their doctor only to then be dismissed because diagnostic tests failed to find anything. The reason for the failure rests on the design of the tests, the purpose of which is to detect disease. Symptoms are often present without a disease. The problem is functional not pathological. Remember, a functional illness is one in which a disruption in any of the body's systems occurs without the presence of a disease. In other words, the body, for whatever reason, is not functioning to its fullest potential and is therefore expending extra nutritional resources in order to maintain homeostasis.

Despite its ability to manage functional illness as demonstrated by its persistent growth, most medical doctors still consider complementary medicine a farce or scam perpetuated on a gullible society. This visceral response is becoming more and more unwarranted, but is not entirely unexpected. No MD wants to go through eight or more years of graduate school, sacrifice a social life and perhaps a family, and accumulate hundreds of thousands of dollars of debt, all to have people tell them their line of thinking and treatment methods are incomplete or perhaps detrimental. The high level of commitment a person dedicates to become a medical doctor guarantees he will be vested: a full-fledged partner in a disease-care system ironically called "healthcare," which results in limited treatment options (drugs and/or surgery) and too often produces arrogant doctors who see the disease model as the only valid approach.

In the disease model, all resources are devoted to the detection and elimination of a definable disease. This may sound good at first. However, if the goal is health, or not getting a disease in the first place, then the philosophy and practice of allopathic medicine is insufficient and limited. If a disease must first be present, by definition, it must mean a person lost their health somewhere along the way. Conversely, **a philosophy of prevention is one that applies resources toward the correction of early-stage imbalances rather than late-stage illnesses and desires to correct imbalances with natural measures rather than address illnesses with unnatural medications.**

Patients are culpable as well, having been willing participants in the generations-long philosophy of pharmaceutical medicine. With hardly a second glance, the masses discarded the ancient wisdom of health and wellness for a get-better-quick-with-a-pill approach and never looked back. In the end their hasty decision has turned out to be one of the most dangerous, wasteful and expensive methods for maintaining health, managing illness and fighting disease.

In the United States, considering all causes of death, medical doctors have the third highest chance of killing someone. Here is the breakdown according to the Journal of the American Medical Association: [151]

- 12,000 deaths annually from unnecessary surgery.

- 7,000 deaths annually from medication errors.

- 20,000 deaths annually from other errors in hospitals.

- 80,000 deaths annually from nosocomial infections (infections acquired in a hospital).

- 106,000 deaths annually from non-error, adverse effects of medications.

"These total to 225,000 deaths per year from iatrogenic causes [resulting from doctors]." These estimates are for deaths only and do not include other adverse effects such as those associated with disability or discomfort.

The article went on to estimate that between 4 and 18 percent of hospital patients experienced adverse effects resulting in the following statistics:

- 116 million extra patient visits.

- 77 million extra prescriptions.

- 17 million emergency department visits.

- 8 million hospitalizations.

- 3 million long-term admissions.

- $77 billion in extra costs.

And this is what so many are fussing about in Congress? Access to a system that has a higher chance of killing a person than diabetes, Alzheimer's, pneumonia and influenza combined?

Japan ranks second only to the United States in the number of advanced diagnostic equipment units, like MRIs and CTs. However, the country ranks highest on health, whereas the United States ranks among the lowest. This seems ironic given the medical technology in the United

States is unsurpassed. How then can the U.S. rank so low on health? The author explains this by noting that American patients diagnosed with an illness are hospitalized, whereas in Japan the common practice is to have the family members provide the amenities of hospital care in the patient's home.

Research has yet to determine all the reasons why home care is statistically better than hospital care. Is it the personal attention? The kindness of family members? The food? The emotional comfort? The reduced risk of infection? Or, some combination? What is clear is that to avoid becoming a statistic like those mentioned above, the best thing to do is to avoid the hospital. And the best way to do that is by avoiding disease. This is what complementary medicine does best; it helps millions around the world recover from the many forms of functional illness and, even in some cases, cancer.[152] [153] Many are beginning to agree with this assessment, which is the reason why complementary medicine has grown robustly year after year. Despite the fact insurance does not cover most complementary care, patients have willingly spent approximately $40 billion out-of-pocket each year. This expensive fact has not gone unnoticed by the traditional medical community.

Rather than offering recognition and acceptance of complementary care, the medical establishment has chosen acquisition and absorption. For example, the evening news aired a special "Health Report" describing an electronic device worn on the wrist to decrease the nausea experienced by cancer patients. The reporter went into great detail explaining how the device worked, touting the wonderful potential benefits. Little did she know it was stimulating a point on an acupuncture meridian well-known for reducing the symptom of nausea. Unfortunately, she didn't use any acupuncture terminology or give the practice credit. To control nausea, acupuncture patients have used similar non-electronic wristbands for years at a cost of around $5.00. This device sold for $150.00.

As a result of demand by satisfied patients, traditional medicine has reluctantly "accepted" some forms of complementary treatment for specific conditions: acupuncture for pain, chiropractic for lower back problems and massage therapy for stress. It is the hope of some practitioners that one day FBA will be among the techniques on the accepted list.

Prior to allopathic doctors extending this olive branch, the only explanation given for treatments that worked but which were not pharmaceutically based was the placebo effect. In other words, the patient so believed he would get better that he often did, through a mysterious process in his own mind. Though the placebo effect is a real phenomenon, it is inadequate as the sole explanation for all the benefits achieved through complementary health care. Interestingly, since complementary health care providers are often the last of many doctors a patient visits for the same condition, doesn't it seem strange the placebo effect took so long to happen? Or, put another way, why didn't the placebo effect occur at the time the medical treatments were given instead of waiting until a complementary treatment was performed?

The fact is standard western medicine is unable to meet the demands of the ever-increasing levels of functional and chronic illness. And how could it? The model of allopathic medicine is to prescribe a drug for a given ailment. Drugs never fix problems; they only force certain reactions to happen at the expense of others, which will then lead to unintended consequences. The role of a drug is to block, inhibit, or down regulate a given biochemical. This approach may have an impact, but it is in no way holistic and cannot bring about homeostasis.

Side effects from medications often require management from a second, third or fourth drug. Pharmaceutical intervention is appropriate in life-threatening situations when the body can no longer help itself and would soon perish. However, these same life-saving drugs, when used for nonlife-threatening illnesses, will make matters much worse, increasing the probability of future chronic illness to a near certainty. This is the current situation for most medicated people.

Where allopathic medicine has reached into the area of prevention, it has often failed. There are no drugs to prevent cancer, only those that attempt to treat it. In fact cancer rates continue to rise. Over the next 20 years, doctors expect the number of new cancer cases diagnosed annually in the United States to increase by 45 percent, from 1.6 million in 2010 to 2.3 million in 2030.[154] There are also no drugs that can prevent heart disease or diabetes. The incidence of the top-ten killers has also increased in recent years with diabetes topping out at 72,000 deaths annually and heart disease reaching a whopping 630,000.[155]

Additionally, drugs are riddled with side effects, including the cholesterol-lowering statin drugs, prescribed for preventative measures.[156] These drugs are very good at lowering cholesterol, but fail to reduce the incidence of heart attacks in those taking them, the purpose for which it was prescribed.[157] If all medical science allows for is the use of synthetic medications for the correction of a natural process, then there is little hope for long-term wellness and vitality via the medical methods. What may work for a temporary aliment or infection will not work with illness and disease, especially when the two are often clustered and interconnected. This is the realm of functional medicine, the area where Functional Bio-Analysis can and does excel.

Reason #2: Finding What Technology Can't

When it comes to functional imbalances, diagnostic tests often fall short. A blood test can determine the level of a given hormone, but can it tell if the body is synthesizing, utilizing and detoxifying the hormone properly? An MRI can reveal an over-worked and enlarged liver, but can it reveal the chemicals ingested in everyday life that the liver is failing to break down? A glucose tolerance test can determine the body is not properly processing sugar, but can it make known which sugar-balancing hormone and which missing minerals are responsible?

The more people learn about functional imbalances, the more researchers realize such imbalances are clustered, multifaceted states. That is, different imbalances are all present at the same time, leaving the body in a seemingly confused and compensatory pattern. Not surprisingly, doctors can't always find the answers they need to circumnavigate the biochemical puzzle in blood, saliva or urine tests. Those two-dimensional snapshots, although extremely important and valuable in their own right, are inadequate investigatory tools for the human body's multidimensional tripartite structure.

The good news is functional imbalances are not random, though it may often appear so. There are reasons why things have regressed to the point they have and why things look as they do. Understanding what is taking place and the significance of the disruptions through Functional Bio-Analysis is at present the most efficient means of health restoration.

When an experienced practitioner who knows the strengths and weaknesses of his craft properly performs FBA, it is one of the most precise, accurate and reliable methods of obtaining metabolic and neurological information. And it does so instantly, inexpensively and without harm—a stark contrast to other forms of diagnosis and treatment. In the years to come, the doctor who can discern, detect and direct the body to recovery and wellness and do so inexpensively and without harm will be worth his weight in platinum.

WHAT COLOR ARE YOU? RED, GREEN, OR BLUE?

Researchers believe genetics hold the key to unlock many of the mysteries of health and disease. They are probably right. Therefore, the more a practitioner knows about the genetics of individuals in need, the better the chances of restoring their health. FBA uses a simple method to broadly categorize patients based on their genetics into one of the three primary colors.

The Three Colors

Light is a waveform. In the year 1666, Isaac Newton used a prism to break visible white light into the rainbow colors of the spectrum, giving impetus to the development of what is now the vast science of optics. Human optics are utterly amazing in their ability to receive and process a wealth of information concerning levels of light intensity, colors, motion and depth of field. Visible light for humans consists of light waves with a wavelength between 400 and 700 nanometers. This range is only one section of the entire electromagnetic spectrum, which permeates the universe with electromagnetic waves that extends from the smallest wavelength found in gamma rays to the largest wavelength found in radio waves. The difference between these ends of the spectrum is at least 16 orders of magnitude.

The smaller the wavelength of light, the more harmful it is to the human body. Ultraviolet rays and X-rays are recognized examples. These light forms are outside of the visible spectrum, but there is also danger within. For instance, scientists have discovered all human beings respond negatively to one of the three primary colors of visible light: red, green and blue. These primary colors are not the same as the primary colors of pigment (red, yellow and blue). From the three colors, the eye can create all other visible colors, much like a projection television combines the light from its three colored lamps to make a movie. However, just any blue won't do. Each of these primary colors has a specific wavelength. The red is 619nm; the green 550nm; and the blue, which looks more like a violet, is 440nm. One of these precise frequencies is harmful to all people by disrupting homeostasis on an energetic level.

The test is easy to carry out. In a well-lit room, the practitioner places each color, one at a time, over both eyes and performs a muscle test. Everyone will weaken to one of the three colors. This simple test, determining which color a person is, can generate a large amount of pertinent health information in only a few seconds. Each of the colors is tied into the genetic makeup of the person and therefore reveals certain tendencies and general health concerns. Detrimental patterns include a major food or class of foods a person should avoid while beneficially indicating certain nutrients that are important for functional health. Much more has been, and is being discovered as well—see the charts below.

Color	Type/General Tendencies	Helpful Nutrition
Red	Heart disease, insulin resistance, diabetes, high blood pressure, high homocysteine	Vitamins B6, B12 & folic acid
Green	Eczema, skin blotchiness, hormonal issues, strong sense of smell, sensitivities to electromagnetic energies such as computers, reactions to nickel jewelry or dental braces	Magnesium sulfate or bromide, liver support, sulfur, evening primrose oil
Blue	Chronic fatigue, joints need to crack/pop, sinus congestion, constipation, hypoglycemia, high cholesterol, growing pains, dental cavities as a child, kidney stones	Calcium, potassium, copper

Color	Foods to Avoid	Good Mineral Types	Metal (poor detoxification)
Red	Wheat	Iodides / Phosphates	Aluminum
Green	Chemicals/ Preservatives	Bromides / Sulfates	Nickel
Blue	Cow-Milk-Based Products	Chlorides	Mercury

With regard to the foods listed above, these are not allergies, they are the opposite. They are agglutination reactions. The difference between allergies and agglutination reactions is that one is fast and the other is slow. Allergies tend to increase immune function and speed up cellular reactions (think runny nose, watery eyes and itchy skin). Whereas, the foods related to the colors cause agglutination, or sticky reactions, slowing things down and making internal processes more sluggish. Agglutination either causes or relates to many dangerous diseases.[158] [159] Detoxification, blood circulation and lymphatic drainage are the first areas hindered by the color-related foods.

As the body expends hormetic nutrients to help with these issues, many other systems experience problems. The body compensates and adapts to the general decline in the overall health level, further using hormetic nutrients. *Eat Right 4 Your Blood Type*, a book by Dr. Peter J. D'Adamo, is an instructive resource that discusses the unique agglutination reactions present in people of different blood types as they eat non-beneficial foods. The colors correlate reasonably well with the different blood types and their general dietary guidelines.

Primary or Secondary Color?

Whichever color weakens a testing-muscle when placed over both eyes is the dominant color, and the one to pay attention to at the moment. But, is it the primary color? Probably not. It is common to have a different color in each eye. The primary color, regardless of whether a person is right- or left-handed, is the color in the left eye. Why the left eye contains the primary color for all people is not known. What is known however, is why the right-eye color shows up first: it is a form of adaptation.

The principle health feature of most is that they survive, not thrive. Compensating to functional imbalances means that life is lived in a state of energy starvation requiring the body to gear down. Movement to a lower energy state is a common adaptive mechanism by the body as it manages the stresses of life. Given that life is a highway, moving along at 65 mph in 1st rather than 3rd gear is bound to have a negative impact – placing undue stress on some systems for the sake of others. When a person moves from their right eye color to their left eye color, health has improved and they have jumped up to third gear. An example may be helpful.

Color testing revealed that a man reacted to blue over both eyes, but to red over his left eye. This means the FBA practitioner should treat the man like a Blue person but not for long. Within a few weeks, as he faithfully takes his hormetic nutrients and follows his doctor's recommendations, the patient should switch colors. Now red over both eyes will weaken a test-muscle. He has moved from 1st to 2nd gear. Getting the body to return to a higher energy state, like with the changing of colors, is a sure sign health is on the way.

Metals and Their Color

There is a very interesting correlation between the metals that the color types should avoid and the spectroscopic analysis of those metals. Spectroscopes break down the light emitted or absorbed by chemical elements into specific lines of color. Astronomers use this instrument to determine the elemental makeup of distance planets and stars. Different elements have their own unique color when evaluated with a spectroscope. Reds, for example, should avoid aluminum. The color of aluminum through spectroscopy is exactly 619nm, the identical frequency that troubles Red people. The same is true for mercury (440nm), the metal that bothers Blues; and nickel (550nm), the disruptive metal for Greens.

Red People (Reds)

Generally those who weaken to the color red are strong body types with strong inner constitutions. They do not tend to get sick easily. However, they are susceptible to heart disease as a result of poor methylation, which is the process of adding a methyl group (CH3) to a compound in order to detoxify or get rid of it. Methylation changes the compound from a free radical into something benign. For instance, the chemical homocysteine directly relates to increased inflammation, the kind that especially affects the cardiac arteries and leads to arteriosclerosis. Red people tend to have trouble with this pesky chemical. Research can directly or indirectly attribute nearly all heart attacks and some other diseases to homocysteine.[160] [161] In fact the smallest increase of homocysteine in the blood can lead to a 20 to 50 percent increase in coronary heart disease risk.[162] Homocysteine is a result of normal metabolic processes but when methylation is poor, the body does not neutralize it. The simple dietary addition of vitamin B12 and/or folic acid, both of which freely donate their methyl groups, could mean the difference between life and premature death. [163] Resolving methylation problems, researchers believe, is one of the most promising approaches to ameliorating genetically-triggered illness.[164]

Reds are also poor detoxifiers of the metal aluminum. As the science mounts, it shows a direct relation between many neurological issues, including Alzheimer's disease, and high levels of this metal in the nervous system.[165,166,167] Consideration for Reds would include avoiding aluminum cookware and foods with aluminum as a preserving agent. This may be harder than it at first seems. Baking powder contains aluminum and is a common ingredient in many processed baked goods such as flour tortillas, pizza crust, muffins, cookies, waffles, etc.

Finally, Reds are the carnivores and require daily dense protein for vitality. Red people should not consider vegetarianism—that would be a double-whammy. Since most B12 comes from meat sources and reds need an above average amount of this vitamin to aid in the breakdown of homocysteine, not eating meat would make them sickly and set them up for a heart attack at the same time.

Green People (Greens)

Greens are chemically sensitive. They are the ones that have the greatest need to eat organically. Perfumes, gasoline, candles and other strong chemical smells are generally very bothersome and cause immediate reactions such as headaches, sneezing and even rashes. One reason for this is Greens tend to have detoxification issues with the liver, specifically sulfation reactions, which require high amounts of the appropriate form of sulfur. Their proper mineral type can be critical to help with this issue as well. Bromides, like magnesium bromide and potassium bromide often provide immediate assistance when a chemical reaction is taking place, as will sulfates such as magnesium sulfate.

In Greens, the body considers environmental and food chemicals to be extremely noxious, and if the liver cannot get rid of them, the skin will. This is why Greens are the ones who tend to get eczema. Practitioners have regularly seen chronic cases of eczema clear up completely just by adding magnesium bromide and sulfur to the daily nutritional regime of Greens. For people who fit into this category, the body will need a dietary balance between proteins and carbohydrates. Healthy portions of organic vegetables are essential for Greens, as well. When it comes to metals, Greens do not easily eliminate nickel. Jewelry and stainless steel are common sources. Greens are the ones who react to cheap jewelry as evidenced by discolorations at the location of skin contact.

Blue People (Blues)

Blues have a more slender body type and are the opposite of "big-boned." They are sensitive to cow milk products. This does not mean they can never have dairy, but they will notice some negative digestive changes, such as constipation, if they do. There are several physical problems that emerge as Blues ingest dairy products. For instance, milk is notorious for causing sinus problems. It does this because of the large amounts of mucous produced with diary consumption and because the sinuses are directly related to the health of the large intestine. Milk products slow down and upset the natural good bacteria in the large intestine of a blue person. This leads to intestinal inflammation, which leads to inflammation in the sinuses.

Blues also have a difficult time managing the large amounts of calcium in milk products. The milk calcium, called calcium lactate, disrupts a blue person's natural calcium balance, leading to one or more ailments such as growing pains and above average dental cavities in childhood. The most significant issue with Blues is their tendency toward hypoglycemia as a result of poor calcium management. Calcium aids the body in the production of glycogen, or stored blood sugar. Without enough of this important substance to fuel the body between meals, blood sugar will crash, initiating a cascade of hormone-altering events discussed in detail in the chapter, *Hypoglycemia or Histamine?*

For metals, mercury is the one Blues do not eliminate well. Mercury is highly toxic and can cause almost any symptom in the body. For diet, Blues are the ones who can get away with a more vegetarian diet. However, in this day and age with blood sugar issues rampant, it would still be very wise to keep protein levels moderate with each meal. Blues do tend to have various ailments on a regular basis and are the ones susceptible to chronic fatigue and fibromyalgia, although these illnesses can happen to any of the color groups.

What's Wrong With Milk and Wheat?

A regular question people raise concerning color-related foods is, why? Wheat and milk are good for people aren't they? Concerning wheat, the protein gluten may be part of the answer. Celiac disease is a destructive, auto-immune, inflammatory reaction in the lower bowels as a result of gluten consumption. Research is linking more than just diseases of the gastro-intestinal tract to this protein, which is found in high levels in wheat products.[168] In populations that introduce gluten at an early age[169] and in those where breast feeding is minimal or not performed, Celiac disease has a higher presence.[170] On the contrary, rates of celiac disease were significantly lower in other populations where the introduction of gluten-containing cereals into the diet of infants was gradual.[171] The second reason why wheat, or any food, can become noxious is related to repeated exposure.

There is no such thing as a perfect food. Everything has its own requirements for digestion and assimilation. The same thing, eaten all the time, means an eventual nutritional deficiency or digestive tissue irritation. Bombardment with the same type of food, processed with the same nutrition-stripping methods will lead to an increase in food-related, functional illness. With foods, the common sense rules of long ago are still in vogue: variety and moderation. There are dozens of varieties of dairy cows and dozens of varieties and cousins of wheat. In America and now around the world, wheat and milk tend to be from sources that can produce these foods the fastest and in the greatest quantity. That always means less nutrition. Sensitive dairy patients often tell practitioners that when they traveled to France and ate the local milk products there, they had no digestive issues at all, whereas they did after eating the same type of food in the U.S. The dairy cows are different in France and certain other countries, and the processing is different (often the dairy is ingested raw without pasteurization).

Milk is a more difficult topic with respect to health. It has an association with Multiple Sclerosis[172] [173] and Type I diabetes.[174] However, milk also seems to be protective for other illnesses such as bladder cancer[175] and colorectal cancer.[176]

As with nearly all illnesses, combinations of factors are at work simultaneously. No one eats only milk products and no one eats only wheat. These foods are always mixed with other foods, making the picture cloudy. Thankfully, with FBA, the view begins to clear. If a person doesn't test well to it, it is best not to do it. Blues never seem to test well to milk. Although they are able to get away with some cheese products (the more aged the better) as can Reds with wheat. The occasional slice of cheddar cheese or a pasta dish, will not send them off a cliff, but rest assured, if dairy or wheat becomes part of the daily routine for Blues or Reds respectively, it will soon drain them of critical nutrients and promote an inflammatory cycle.

BODY BASICS

FBA is a step-by-step, point-by-point analysis and correction of the body performed in the manner already predetermined by the brain. There are 15 primary energetic points (PEP). Each of these points corresponds to an organ or a system. Liver 14 (LV14) for instance relates to the functions of the liver. Circulation Sex 1 (CX1) pairs with the entire system that governs reproductive hormones. A standard analysis with FBA will lead the practitioner through the layers of need. Four or five layers are common for most people. Each layer relates to one of the 15 reflex points and will require just one hormetic nutrient to bring it back to homeostasis (some layers may require two).

In order to gather the appropriate data for health restoration, FBA is dependent upon manual muscle testing (MMT). The test-muscle used for the analysis is usually an arm or leg muscle depending upon doctor and patient comfort. MMT should never be a struggle. A low to moderate amount of force is all that is required. Anything more indicates that something is wrong, such as a previous injury. A previously injured muscle will likely not respond with the appropriate sensitivity and requires special treatments in order to overcome the neurological issues that arise from an injury. Therefore, it is always best to use a test muscle that is injury-free.

So, what can FBA treat? All problems, conditions, illnesses and diseases result in, or are the result of, nutritional imbalances. Since FBA is designed to search for the nutrients the body needs most, anyone, no matter what his or her current health state, can benefit. Does this mean that FBA cures cancer? No, it wouldn't be prudent to say that (although, hormetic nutrients and botanicals are being studied for their cancer-killing effects).[177] [178] FBA does help cancer patients tremendously as an adjunct while they are undergoing chemotherapy or radiation therapy. What FBA can, and often does cure, is detailed in the chapters that follow.

FBA practitioners navigate the energetic pathway of the body looking for the body's most needed nutrients. Using these hormetic nutrients to balance neurotransmitters and hormones is one of the most effective ways to correct functional illnesses and restore health. Why? Because fixing these major components of human physiology restores not only local disruptions, but global body rhythms as well.

HORMETIC NUTRIENTS – DOING THE MOST WITH THE LEAST

Finding hormetic nutrients is the main goal of FBA. Remember, a hormetic nutrient will positively impact multiple systems simultaneously. Finding these is the most efficient means of breaking disease-promoting cycles and correcting physiological imbalances. Any nutrient - magnesium, calcium, B vitamins, oils, anti-oxidants have the potential to produce a hormetic effect. So do botanicals and the compounds within them.

Botanicals, the medicines of nature, are plant-based substances made up of thousands of compounds. Herbs, barks, leaves, roots, fruits, seeds and even spices all have a healing role to play. Examples include: panex ginseng, rhodiola, curcumin, echinacea and ashwaganda. The potential of most botanicals has not been fully realized and, it is likely, the health-rendering properties of many others are yet to be discovered. The more chronic a condition the more likely a balancing botanical may be necessary to initiate healing.

Hormetic nutrients are used up rapidly during times of stress. The result is a plethora of nutritional potholes. Through a triage mechanism, the body allocates the use of nutrients in a manner that favors short-term survival at the expense of long-term health.[179] Most people therefore, are deficient in one or more nutrients, but their deficiencies are not the same. A nutrient may be hormetic for one person, but do nothing for the next. Magnesium for example, is required in seventy percent of all enzymes— the catalyzing proteins that make biochemistry happen rapidly. It will only however, have a hormetic effect in the person who has a magnesium deficiency, not in one who doesn't.

Finding out whether or not a nutrient is hormetic is the job of FBA. Navigating the body's energetic roadmap often uncovers four or five hormetic nutrients. These all work together to fix the same number of systems. Some additional functions of hormetic nutrients include the following:

- Producing energy,[180] [181] [182]
- Regulating genetic expression,[183] [184] [185] [186]
- Activating enzymes,[187] [188] [189]
- Controlling inflammation,[190] [191] [192] [193]
- Detoxifying tissues,[194] [195]
- Regulating metabolism,[196] [197] [198]
- Regulating blood pressure,[199] [200] [201] [202]
- Regulating emotional stress and neurotransmitters,[203] [204] [205] [206]
- Balancing hormones,[207] [208] [209] [210]
- Slowing down the aging process[211] [212]
- And controlling pain levels.[213] [214] [215]

This list above includes many of the most common patient complaints. The origin of these and other functional problems is not mysterious. Most start with diet. Traumas, ongoing infections, emotional stresses and genetics are also important considerations. Collectively, these concerns promote a vicious energy-exhausting cycle and lead a person on a pathway toward disease through unwanted genetic expression.[216] Keeping genes in check is the job of the hormetic nutrients.

At present, roughly 50 different human genetic diseases arise when the wrong mutant enzymes replace the right B-vitamins, called coenzymes. This disease-promoting situation is set up when proper levels of B-vitamins are too low, and it can be remedied when those levels are high. Raising the levels therefore prevents unwanted gene expression, called polymorphisms,[217] the source for many known diseases.

The civilized diet is the greatest reason why health is initially disrupted. After ingesting food, a healthy body utilizes what it requires, stores what it needs for later use, and eliminates what is unnecessary. When there are no hiccups in this process, it acquires and stores hormetic nutrients throughout life as individuals eat the right foods and avoid the wrong ones. However, the high ingestion of nutrient-stripping processed foods found in the modern diet eventually means hiccups are more the rule than the exception. There are other considerations, as well.

FBA practitioners believe in an interconnected and interrelated set of systems that work together to promote the optimal expression of well-being. None of these systems is greater than the other, but each can move to the front of the line depending on the stresses of the moment. In other words, **there is a hierarchy within the major systems of the body and the body's most pressing needs are at the top.** With any number of circumstances, the main concern can change. For instance, a sudden event such as a motor vehicle accident, which results in muscle and joint trauma, could make the musculoskeletal system a top priority. The sudden fear of losing a job or the death of a loved one could make the emotional system a top priority. A weekend binge on junk food and alcohol could make the chemical system a top priority. However, in "normal" life, where stress is somewhat constant and slower to mount up, it is more often the chemical system that requires the most attention.

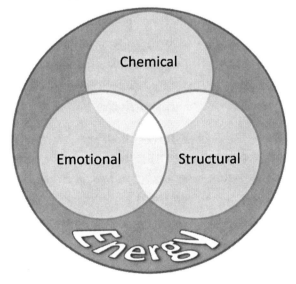

Figure 3: Body and Energy

Each of the three major physical systems depends on a constant steady supply of energy. If energy is not flowing properly through the body from organ to organ and from system to system, health issues will manifest. The management and proper flow of energy is the goal of many non-traditional techniques such as acupuncture, tai chi, homeopathy and even laser therapy. Their popularity is partial evidence of their validity. Knowing this, many patients and practitioners have concluded energy management is the most important consideration for health. That could be, and often is, true, but the underlying assumption is that there is plenty of internal energy to go around. However, what happens if the total energy in the body is low? Energy therapies are not involved in energy creation, but rather energy utilization and management. So, the pertinent question is, where does energy come from in the human body?

Since humans do not photosynthesize like plants, it is not from the sun, although sunlight is very important for overall health. It is not from muscles or bones, although movement through exercise is critical for overall wellbeing. It is not from thoughts, although thinking good thoughts and having an overall positive outlook is helpful. The principle source of energy production is via nutrients contained within foods. In other words, **energy comes from chemistry**. Common sense confirms this is true. Exercising in the sunlight while listening to motivational speakers on an iPod will likely have some health benefits, but even the healthiest, most stress-relieving practices will prove to be in vain without proper food. Failing to consume the correct nutrients allows life (energy) to gradually dissipate.

Just eating any food won't do—Americans eat plenty of food. Nearly 34 percent of adults are obese; more than double the percentage 30 years ago. The share of obese children tripled during that time, to 17 percent.[218] And yet, nutritional deficiencies are still widespread. No, most people are not exhibiting signs of pellagra, rickets or scurvy, but what they are doing is managing a cluster of issues that, as a whole, prevent them from expressing optimal function. This is so because nutrition determines chemistry, and chemistry determines function. Functional illnesses therefore, are primarily the result of chemical problems. In addition, where the chemical problems are located (in the brain for instance) can often determine the severity of the problem.

Some people think they don't have any chemical problems. They are almost certainly wrong. Aging is a chemical problem and you and I have yet to meet someone who doesn't age. Beyond this universal example, as a regular part of life, the person who experiences pain, insomnia, constipation, fatigue, headaches, PMS or emotional issues such as depression or anxiety, has chemical problems. If they admit things like, "I just have a bad back (knees, hips, etc.)," or, "I get up twice a night to go to the bathroom, but that is normal." They have chemical problems. If taking over-the-counter pain, stomach or allergy medication is a common practice, they have chemical problems. In short, if the regular experience of life is anything other than a pain-free, passion-filled existence, that person has chemical problems.

A QUICK LOOK AT DIET

He who takes medicine and neglects to diet wastes the skill of his doctors. ~ *Chinese Proverb*

Food determines the quality and quantity of essential nutrients. If the ingoing chemicals are bad, the internal energy eventually is poor, causing the overall function of the body to decline. Hormetic nutrients direct the internal chemistry of the body and optimally should come from the diet. Therefore, eating well is critical to proper function.

According to the United States Department of Agriculture (USDA), more than 70 percent of men and women eat less than two-thirds of the Recommended Daily Intake (RDI) for one or more nutrients[219] and only 10 percent of the American population eats five or more servings of fruits and vegetables per day. In other words, the Standard American Diet (SAD) is saturated with low-nutrient, fatty foods comprised of empty calories and little nutritional value. Today, American consumers spend 90 percent of their typical food bill on nutrient-void processed foods.[220]

The Industrial Revolution led to the introduction of sucrose (white sugar), mass-produced meats, refined grains, refined vegetable oils, hydrogenated oils and high fructose corn syrup (HFCS). It also created ways of extracting oils and nutrients from foods in order to extend the shelf-life, which made it possible to transport foods across great distances without spoilage. However, what was good for convenience and mass consumption was not good for physiology, as these processes greatly diminished, or stripped out completely, the natural hormetic nutrients and replaced them with synthetic versions. Synthetic vitamins may help prevent gross nutritional deficiencies, but the dosage required is much greater than that found in nature and, in some cases, they initiate biochemical imbalances.[221] [222]

Worse yet, many foods are also genetically modified (GM or GMO). The modifications produce greater yields, help plants resist bugs and protect food from potent insecticides and herbicides. Unlike the selective breeding and farming done since the beginning to encourage desirable traits, scientists are tinkering with the genetic code of foods and animals with some very unpleasant results. Instead of using nature to bring about the healthiest and most productive crops, scientists have delved into a world so complicated it is difficult to even imagine.

Modifying food crops means tampering with a plants genetic material. In plants, genes determine things like height, color, leaf size, fruit size and growth rate. But how do each of these individual genes work together for the health of the entire plant? Like a group of football players, each has a specific position on the field and a particular role to play, but what determines their success is how they work as a team. Scientists have little understanding of genetic teamwork in plants or people. What they do know, is that adding and subtracting genes in the laboratory regularly generates surprises and unintended consequences such as increasing the toxins in yeast 40 to 200 times, generating new toxins in tobacco plants where they never existed before and elevating the starch content in potatoes.[223] This means that an individual gene affected more than a single trait, but had a systemic consequence as well. Researchers may take pride in creating a chemical-resistant food crop, one that when sprayed with insecticides and herbicides will kill everything in the field except the plant itself; however, common sense screams that serving Frankenstein-foods for dinner is a recipe for monsters and nightmares.

In addition to nutrition, stress is the second reason for low levels of hormetic nutrients. Assuming children are raised in a wholesome emotional environment, their total level of stress is minimal. Children do not have jobs, manage finances, balance complex relationships, are not sleep deprived, are not seeking to advance their careers and are not concerned with world events or fighting political outrages. They are just children. Aging, adulthood and awareness bring about the emotional, physical and chemical stresses of life. The greatest stress on children is what goes into their mouths. Cereal and milk for breakfast, peanut butter and jelly washed down with fruit juice or soda for lunch, candy or cookies for a snack with a glass of milk, chicken fingers or macaroni and cheese for dinner, is a common menu in most homes. Children can get away with this lifeless fare because hormetic nutrients keep digestion working well. Adults who eat this diet for a week will need a laxative or antacid. And yet, children eat this way from age 2 to 20.

As children grow into puberty, a great hormonal change (stress) begins taking place. This change, along with the chemical stresses of their poor diet, begins to add up. Acne and other skin issues, stomach aches, random muscle or joint pain, headaches, PMS and sleep issues are the common complaints of adolescence. The hormetic nutrients should manage these "normal" experiences of the teenage years, but when their reserves run low, their effectiveness begins to wane.

The ideal diet then would be full of whole, unprocessed foods. Natural whole foods contain not only macro-nutrition in the form of fats, carbohydrates and proteins, but also micro-nutrition such as enzymes and hormetic nutrients. Micro-nutrition is essential in all food, since it is the catalyst of digestion, speeding up the entire process and saving energy. Many people wonder how it is they now have nutritional deficiencies when their entire lives they have "been fine." There is no such thing as a perfect food, and many of the staple foods of today are quite imperfect.

Eating low-nutrition foods devoid of hormetic nutrients strains the digestive process. Since they are not present in the poor quality food itself, hormetic nutrients must come from the internal reserves. Much like the debt-based society Americans live in today, the body has borrowed and borrowed until there is not enough left even to pay the interest. With the regular consumption of processed, low-nutrient and perhaps GMO foods, the body's bank account of hormetic nutrients is spent to satisfy its daily entitlements. The result is a systemic nutritional deficiency.

7 RULES FOR SUPPLEMENTS – MAKING SURE THEY WORK

Nutritional supplementation has a demonstrated effectiveness for a variety of ailments[224] [225] [226] and consequently has led to a multi-billion dollar vitamin industry. According to the Council for Responsible Nutrition, around 40 percent of all people in the U.S. and a majority of woman over age 50 are taking some form of dietary supplementation.[227] Proof of its popularity is visible in gyms, grocery stores and even gas stations, where supplements are readily available. In urban areas, stand-alone vitamin stores are common place containing floor-to-ceiling displays of all the latest and greatest products. Here is where the confusion sets in: Given the number of possibilities right before their eyes, how can consumers, even knowledgeable ones, know which version of a product is right for them? Certainly the vitamins cannot all be the same. The best a consumer can do is to make her choice based upon quality and perhaps research. But there is more; much more. Presented below are the seven reasons why supplementation may have no beneficial effect whatsoever. The first two are generally recognized. The last five, however, are ones many in the world of alternative medicine do not even know.

Rule #1: Is It What It Says It Is and Nothing Else?
The quality and purity of any ingested product is a chief concern for consumers and is one of the main regulatory assignments of the Food and

Drug Administration. Unfortunately, what is on the label is not always what is in the package.

In a University of Maryland Pharmacy School study in 2000, only 2 of 32 different joint supplements (containing chondroitin sulfate) met the label claim for ingredients. The study reported the less expensive the supplement, the lower the total levels of the nutrient.[228] Unfortunately, several similar studies have been performed on a variety of different types of supplements, only to find analogous results.[229] [230]

Another concern with supplements is their overall quality. Despite claims of purity on the label, as a percentage, very few companies actually measure up. Poor quality means a product full of binders, fillers and lubricants. Magnesium sterate, ascorbyl palmitate, lactose and sodium benzoate are just a few examples. These cost-cutting and production-assisting additives can lead to poor absorption and potential allergic reactions. Beyond this, the methods of preparation and storage of raw materials is very important to avoid potential contaminants such as molds, bacteria or heavy metals.

Rule #2: Is It What People Need With Nothing Else?

Each person is unique. This means that supplements, even ultra-pure supplements, might work for one person but not for others. Just because vitamin C is good to help the immune system, does not mean it is good in every case. In fact, depending upon the type of immune system imbalance, it could actually make things worse.

Similarly, metabolism, like genetics, is personal. But unlike genetics, metabolism is highly dynamic and can change based on diet, stress, lack of rest, increased or decreased activity and more. This adds to the confusion concerning how long to take a given supplement, and it is the reason why nutrients that used to work are no longer effective. Therefore, a regular evaluation of one's current supplement regime is critical.

Rule #3: Multi-Vitamins Are For Healthy People

Recognizing that extra nutrients are needed in the diet, a large percentage of people have become proactive, even religious, by taking a multi-vitamin. The assumption is a once-a-day multiple vitamin containing B-vitamins, minerals, antioxidants and the latest wild berry plucked from an isolated rock outcropping in Papua New Guinea will meet the nutritional needs of the body. If only it were that easy. For those with functional illness, just taking a multi-vitamin will probably not work. In the case of autoimmunity, it could even get worse. Multiple vitamins are only effective for healthy people or those who are severely nutritionally deprived.[231] The reason why multi-vitamins are ineffective, even detrimental, has everything to do with the next rule.

Rule #4: Anything Can Be Canceled Out or Neutralized

It is not surprising for FBA practitioners to see a patient carry a large box of supplements into the office and then crash it on to their desk. As soon as this happens, good practitioners know they are about to be a hero. In some cases, it is possible to take the patient off of half to two-thirds of his supplements, while seeing his health improve at the same time. Most vitamin collectors are well informed and have made wise choices based upon the latest eBlast from a respected alternative health doctor or vitamin store. Yes, everything they are taking is of good quality, and the latest research "proves" the supplements have positive health benefits. But, it is the simple case of too much of a good thing becoming a bad thing. Researchers do not conduct studies with patients taking ten or more nutrients at the same time. This would be bad science. Yet, too many nutrients equal too much internal processing. It is hard to fix one internal stress by creating another.

For example, a patient may complain of extended soreness after exercise. This is often a need for vitamin B1, which the muscles use to break down lactic acid. The same patient may complain of chronic allergies. This is often a need for vitamin B6, which is important for metabolizing histamine. So, why not give him a B-complex that has plenty of vitamin B1 and plenty of vitamin B6? Because it probably won't work. Vitamins compete with vitamins, and minerals compete with minerals. Oils compete with oils, and amino acids compete with amino acids. They all can potentially cancel each other out. This is the Teeter-Totter Effect. Finding the precise nutrient and giving that alone, without interference from others, is what makes miracles happen.

Rule #5: Everything Is On a Teeter-Totter

A balance between essential nutrients is critical for optimal function. Most (perhaps all) hormetic nutrients in the body are balanced with another hormetic nutrient. If one is too low, the other, by relative relationship, will be too high. This, as described earlier, is the Teeter-Totter Effect. Trying to use a multi-vitamin to raise up the low side of the teeter-totter almost never works since a multi-vitamin, by definition, will also contain the high or opposite nutrient as well. More on this topic is presented in the section below, *Biorhythms & Teeter-Totters*.

Rule #6 – As The Body Changes, So Do Supplements

When new patients undergo Functional Bio-Analysis, practitioners often find a majority of the patients' shopping-bags-worth of supplements don't do any good. Some are detrimental to a certain tissue, while others are in fact toxic to the body as a whole, causing some of the complaints that brought the patients into the office in the first place. When questioned about the length of time they have been taking their supplements, "years" is not an uncommon answer. Just as there is no perfect food, there is no perfect supplement. Nothing should ever be taken for years. That is because the body is always in a state of change, adapting to life's many stresses. With changes in life there are changes in needs.

When correcting problems with hormetic nutrients, positive changes can happen in weeks. Therefore, supplements should change, or the patient should no longer need them, after only a short period of time. Hormetic nutrients are not just Band-Aids, they correct problems. If a person needs the same supplements for extended periods of time and the problem is not getting fixed, something was missed. The only time a patient will need supplemental nutrients for the long-term is when he is addressing genetic issues or when he is in the middle of an ongoing stressful situation or event with no immediate end in sight.

Rule # 7 – Fixing Chronic Problems is Unnatural

"My supplement is made from organic whole food ingredients like those found in nature" is the argument by both patients and practitioners. On paper, these forms of supplements sound like the best things to take to restore health. Unfortunately, they often are not. Or, if they do work, they require massive doses (and expense) and a "healing crisis" to produce results. Medicines are based on chemicals found in plants, but in an isolated form, making them much more potent than when they were combined with other ingredients in their natural state. This is a clue. The more pure, or isolated, a substance, the more powerful its effect. In other words, purity equals potency. Hormetic nutrients, when properly given, often produce the same clinical potency as medicines, but without the harmful side-effects.

The more severe or chronic problems are, the greater the nutritional deficiencies will be and the more likely it is that hormetic nutrients need to be used all by themselves. As mentioned above, trying to treat significant nutritional imbalances with multiple vitamins almost never works. In severe cases, an imbalance must be treated with an imbalance. Echinacea is a good immune-supporting herb that has helped many to overcome general viral and bacterial illnesses. However, with a raging infection, choose an antibiotic instead. In other words, choose the unnatural, single use, purified, high dosage, out-of-balance option over the general use, complex-chemical, naturally balanced one. Or, better yet, find out through FBA which part of the immune system is in greatest need and supplement it specifically with what is missing to produce the same healing effect as an antibiotic without the gastro-intestinal and common allergic side-effects.

These seven rules are the scientific reality of supplemental nutrition and the experience of those using FBA with their patients. Supplement overload is the reason why many in the alternative field, who are doing things naturally, still fail to help those in need. Understanding and applying these rules with the immediate feedback generated through FBA to find hormetic nutrients, equals fewer supplements, less money, quicker responses and lasting results.

BALANCING HORMONES

Balancing hormones is one of the principal applications of FBA. To do this, an understanding of how hormones are turned on and off is required. A small tissue bundle on the bottom side of the brain called the pituitary gland regulates most hormones. To keep them at proper levels, the body makes hormones based upon a negative feedback loop. For instance, if a woman is low in estrogen, the pituitary gland will release another hormone called follicle stimulating hormone (FSH), which will stimulate the adrenal glands and the ovaries and encourage them to make more estrogen. If her estrogen is too high, the pituitary stops releasing FSH, and estrogen naturally drops as the liver breaks it down. Negative feedback loops are common in everyday life. When the house gets too cold, the thermostat "tells" the furnace to start working. Once the house is warm, the thermostat stops talking, and the furnace no longer makes any heat. The house is similar to the human body: The thermostat is the pituitary gland, and hormones are the heat.

A healthy pituitary gland is constantly turning on and off, regulating the hormonal system in a steady, rhythmic fashion. Wild swings in hormones are a big stress for this gland. Too little hormone for prolonged periods means the pituitary is working overtime, while too much hormone for long periods means the pituitary doesn't work enough. This straightforward feedback of hormone regulation is beautiful in design and function but is also somewhat fragile and easily influenced. There are three common patterns of functional disturbance related to the hormonal system.

Pituitary Slumber – The Hormone House is Too Cold

Pituitary slumber is a regular occurrence resulting from eating too many refined sweeteners. Sugary foods cause surges of insulin, which has a drugging effect and lulls the pituitary to sleep as the body tries to manage a sweet-food surplus. Cortisol from the adrenal glands soon follows to counterbalance the high insulin levels and further suppresses pituitary function. In this state, the pituitary gland does not respond by stimulating endocrine tissues when hormones are low. Poor hormonal rhythm and blood sugar swings are the consequence. Corrections for this condition are detailed in the chapter *Hypoglycemia or Histamine?*

Pituitary Suppression – The Hormone House is Too Hot

If the house is always hot, the thermostat never needs to tell the furnace to make heat. This may not matter to the inanimate thermostat, but it matters greatly to living tissue like the pituitary gland. *Use it or lose it* applies here. If the pituitary gland is not regularly involved in life's rhythmic processes, it loses tone and begins to atrophy. This happens when there is too much hormone available.

Remember, once the body makes something, it must use it or break it down. This, for the most part, is the responsibility of the liver. Beginning in adolescence and encouraged by a sweets-and-grease diet, poor liver detoxification leads to excess hormone levels, especially in young women. All PMS symptoms, including cramps, breast tenderness, irritability, and headaches, directly relate to the inability of a woman to fully metabolize and break down estrogen, progesterone, or one of their subtypes. The entire process is further agitated by the unwarranted and prolonged use of birth control pills, which are usually an artificial form of estrogen. This topic is covered in detail in the chapter *Happy or Hormonal?*

Bio-identical hormone replacement therapy (HRT) is the second method that creates excess hormone and causes a state of pituitary suppression. This condition of hormonal abundance guarantees that the house becomes too hot, leading to a suppressed pituitary gland. Doctors often prescribe HRT when hormone levels in the body are low, as when women are in menopause or perimenopause. HRT is like using space heaters when the furnace is broken. This is an appropriate short-term usage. However, space heaters are not under the influence of the thermostat, and leaving them on all night can be uncomfortable or even dangerous. Long-term use of hormone replacement leads to a dependence upon artificial hormone regulation and promotes a nasty situation called hormone resistance.

Hormones change how cells function. If a cell is constantly bombarded by hormones, it becomes over stimulated. This is an unhealthy state for the cell and the body as a whole. The receptor sites where hormones attach are like the cell's ears, hearing and responding to the hormonal commands. Too many hormones, like too much talking at the same time, soon becomes a bothersome noise. To protect against this state, cells do what they must by cutting off their own ears. As much as 90 percent of receptors can be missing in those with genetic abnormalities.[232] [233]

Those experiencing hormonal resistance are in bad shape. They have too many hormones talking, but no one is listening. To further complicate the matter, in the state of hormone resistance, too much of a hormone produces the exact same outward symptoms as too little. For example, someone with hormone resistance who has too much serotonin may still suffer from depression in the same way as someone with too little. Even though the necessary serotonin is present, the body is not responding to it. It has gone deaf. Treating a patient based solely upon their symptoms will often mean prescribing a medicine or nutrient for one state, when the body needs exactly the opposite. Thankfully, testing with FBA reveals the precise state of the hormone and the exact hormetic nutrient needed to balance it.

Pituitary Stimulation – Too Hot, Too Cold

It is possible that the pituitary gland begins to behave outside of the normal negative feedback loop, making the hot hotter and the cold colder. This is a dangerous situation that produces extreme and often debilitating symptoms. Traumas and congenital abnormalities are the two disease-related reasons for a rogue pituitary gland. From a functional perspective, however, only one reason exists: heavy metal toxicity. Greens, those who are especially sensitive to chemicals of all sorts including heavy metals, are the most susceptible to this unwanted disturbance. The topic of heavy metals is covered in detail in the chapter *Migraines, Metals, or Minerals?*

BIORHYTHMS & TEETER-TOTTERS

The inescapable fact is that all life is replete with and governed by cycles. Man lives according to his inward bodily cycles and according to outward celestial cycles:

> *And God said, "Let there be lights in the firmament of the heaven to divide the day from the night; and let them be for signs, and for seasons, and for days, and years."* Genesis 1:14

Perhaps the two most studied and well-recognized human cycles are the daily and monthly cycles. The daily cycle, called the circadian rhythm, governs the sleep and wake cycle, while the monthly cycle, called the menstrual cycle, governs the monthly rhythm of female hormones. If any chemical substances could be said to be in charge of the inward cycles, it would be hormones. Interaction between these powerful protein molecules should create rhythm, which is why all body cycles are called biorhythms. Disruption of the normal physiological ebb and flow is a sign of functional illness and a cause of future disease. Therefore, the intentional preservation and maintenance of biorhythms should be a top priority when attempting to advance health.

A body without internal rhythm is an accident waiting to happen. Disordered biorhythms relate to poor memory,[234] increased breast cancer rates in women[235] and increased cardiovascular disease.[236] They promote hypoglycemia and metabolic syndrome[237] and are the primary reason for mood disturbances, such as depression.[238]

All the organs of the body have their own internal clock. There are 12 major organs or systems, and each has a special two-hour time slot. This is the time when the body provides the organs with an additional boost of energy in order to do some extra housecleaning. For instance, liver-time is between the hours of 1 a.m. and 3 a.m. This is the most common time for people to awaken during the night. If the evening meal or bedtime snack was especially junky, those with already over-worked livers can expect a wakeup call between these hours. The call will most likely come in the form of a vivid dream or a nightmare. Lung-time is between 3 a.m. and 5 a.m. Those with respiratory problems often wake during these hours. Small children with upper respiratory infections will likely have coughing fits during this time, as well.

Disruption of the body clock happens easily under prolonged stress; under the influence of artificial light, such as when staying up late watching television or working on the computer; by working the night shift; or when crossing several time zones. A person can use simple techniques to rebalance the normal energy flow and "tap" the body back into the proper time. These techniques are powerful but have no permanent effect if the person fails to change his or her lifestyle.

Restoring proper sleep patterns is the best way to begin balancing abnormal circadian rhythms. Deep, restful sleep is dependent upon several factors, but a critical one is the rhythm between two hormones: cortisol and melatonin. The outer part of the adrenal gland makes cortisol, and melatonin is a downstream product of serotonin. Each of these important hormones is discussed at length in later sections. Concerning sleep, cortisol must be at high levels in the morning and at low levels at night. Melatonin is just the opposite. It increases at night when things get dark. The absence of light causes a gland in the brain called the pineal gland to become active, encouraging additional melatonin production. Simply turning the lights down to low levels and intentionally going to sleep before 10 p.m. can help a great deal. The figure below shows what the normal pattern between cortisol and melatonin should look like.

Normal Circadian Rhythm

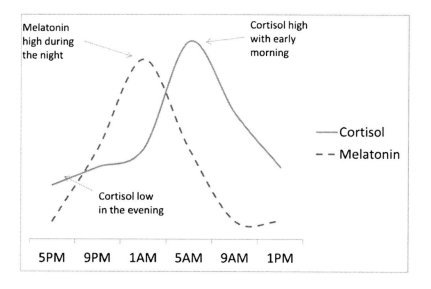

Figure 4: Normal Circadian Rhythm

As one might guess, this is not the pattern of most people with functional problems. They are much more likely to have an abnormal circadian rhythm. This means the levels of cortisol are the inverse of what they should be, while melatonin never reaches a sufficient level for deep sleep. Signs related to disrupted circadian rhythms include the inability to fall asleep or stay asleep, difficulty waking up in the morning, not feeling rested after sleep, a drop in energy between 4 and 7 p.m., and headaches in a daytime, or what is called a diurnal pattern.

Abnormal Circadian Rhythm

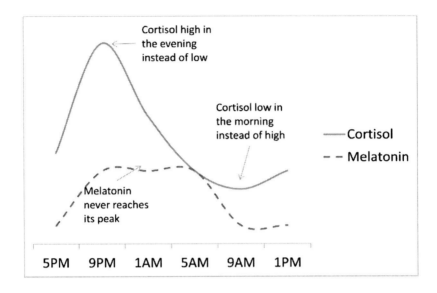

Teeter-Totters

Non-cyclic balance in the body is just as important for health maintenance as cyclic biorhythms. Just as there are hormones pushing and pulling each other in a cyclic fashion, entire systems of the body and individual nutrients do the same thing but in non-cyclic manner. Their give and take looks more like the action of a teeter-totter. When a non-cyclic imbalance is a disruptor of health, the phenomenon is called the Teeter-Totter Effect. Fewer symptoms and a higher level of function are the result of balanced teeter-totters. Below is a list of common teeter-totter pairs regularly evaluated with FBA:

- Serotonin and Dopamine.
- Estrogen and Progesterone.
- The immune system (TH-1 vs. TH-2).
- The nervous system (sympathetic vs. parasympathetic).
- Calcium and Vitamin D.
- Calcium and Magnesium.

- Iron, Zinc and Copper (a three-way teeter-totter).

- Vitamins B1 and B2.

- Sodium and Potassium.

When symptoms of any kind are present, it is likely the Teeter-Totter Effect is in play. For example, serotonin and dopamine, two neurotransmitters essential for proper brain function, are on the same teeter-totter. If serotonin is high, dopamine will most often be low, and vice versa. Migraine headaches, for example, are a sign of too much serotonin in the brain. However, "too much" is relative to dopamine. Therefore, a person suffering from migraines could have high serotonin with normal dopamine levels. Or, he or she could have normal serotonin with low dopamine levels. Either way, the teeter-totter looks the same, and the migraine symptoms are the same. However, in one case the goal is to lower serotonin, while in the other case, the goal is to raise dopamine (sometimes a person will need both). Choosing the wrong treatment will have no effect or could even make things worse.

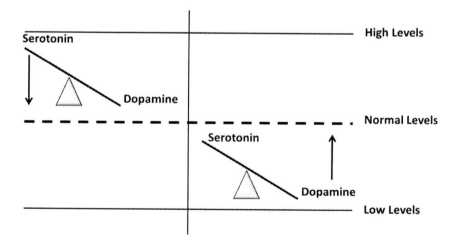

Figure 5: Types of Teeter-Totters

At present, no diagnostic test is available through traditional medicine that can inform a patient as to whether he or she has high, normal or low serotonin. It is an educated guess. FBA, however, can correctly identify the problem. Simply by exposing the patient to a sample of the neurotransmitter serotonin and evaluating the response via the muscles, a practitioner can obtain an instant data point and determine the direction the teeter-totter needs to move. Understanding biorhythms and teeter-totters is extraordinarily helpful to the FBA practitioner as he follows the body's revealed hierarchy, searching for the best hormetic nutrients to restore health. Before FBA testing can begin and be reliable, the practitioner must prepare the patient's body for testing.

GETTING THE BODY READY

Manual Muscle Testing (MMT), in any of its forms, is not perfect. FBA is no exception. The goal of FBA is to tap into the body's own natural monitoring system in order to evaluate energetic reflexes and small samples of various substances. This electromagnetic monitoring system is present in all people but doesn't mean communication between the doctor and patient's body is always immediate. Some preliminary in-office corrections are often necessary before initiating MMT.

The good news is practitioners of FBA understand the obstacles, which are easy to overcome in many cases. Muscle testing should never be a struggle between doctor and patient. A low to moderate amount of force is all it should require. Anything more indicates the body is attending to other issues. In other words, it is distracted. The body will not hear whispers at rock concerts. The smell of flowers in a field dissipates on a windy day. The surrounding world is lost when concentrating on a good book, as is the light touch of soft pajamas after putting on a heavy robe. All sorts of stimuli (sights, sounds, smells, etc.) are discernable, but the more stimulation present or the greater the focus on a single stimulant the less the body will consciously notice others.

Because there is so much the body must pay attention to and the conscious realm cannot express them all, it is more often the exception than the rule that patients are not ready at a moment's notice to have their muscles tested. In FBA, the sensitive energetic reflexes along with small amounts of various biochemical substances such as hormones, neurotransmitters, minerals or foods are the things that need to be tested the most. A body that is medicated, injured or emotionally overwhelmed does not pay attention to these small stimuli. It is not operating in a sensitive enough "mode" to make it testable with MMT. It is too busy dealing with bigger problems. It is too busy dealing with stress.

When people think of stress, they think first of the emotional strain that comes from a bad work environment, struggling relationships, worries over finances or concerns for an ailing loved one. Stress is this and much more. **Stress, for FBA purposes, is anything that shifts the body off balance resulting in an exaggerated biochemical response in order to right itself back into homeostasis.** This means an injury is a stress, requiring the immune system to activate to heal damaged tissue. Medications cause stress, because the liver and the kidneys must detoxify them. A mind overrun with thoughts and a body without enough rest, water or exercise are also forms of stress. The more accumulated stress on the body the more the adrenaline-based survival response, known as "fight-or-flight," overruns other basic functions. This means the response confiscates resources set aside for general wellbeing and directs them toward survival. When the fight-or-flight response becomes part of regular life instead of a short-term change to escape a temporary problem, health and wellness are not possible. Sadly, this is the state in which most people in modern society find themselves. Relieving the fight-or-flight burden is one of the healthiest things any doctor can do.

Preparing a patient for muscle testing is not difficult. There are simple in-office techniques that can reduce the overall stress load and relax and calm the nervous system to the point where muscle testing becomes reliable and accurate. These techniques free the brain/body from survival management, thereby allowing an evaluation of more subtle electromagnetic signals. There are many ways to do this. Any relaxation technique, even those using light and sound, can be effective. The quickest way to reduce the overall stress burden is to realign and rebalance the structure through spinal, pelvic, muscular and cranial bone manipulations. Chiropractors, cranial sacral therapist and other manual therapists utilize these techniques. The effectiveness of this method occurs because of the structure's role as a storage place for excess stress.

Stress in the structure is a well-recognized phenomenon. Patients often grab the back of their neck and with a wincing face declare, "This is where I store my stress." In a large sense, they're right. Any internal chemical or emotional problem will have a structural manifestation. This is the foundational concept upon which many MMT techniques are built. The structure imbalance is generally the last thing to show up in these cases and is the first thing to get better. This is the reason why many think they don't have chemical problems (because they don't currently hurt) and why others have aches, pains and degenerating joints without ever injuring or over-exerting themselves. A person can see this reality simply by looking in the mirror. Most right-handed people will have a lower right shoulder when compared to the left. They will also have a higher right hip. The opposite pattern is true for left-handed people. This common postural misalignment results from the body managing internal stresses through external structure.

In the office, spending a few minutes realigning the misaligned cranial and spinal segments is usually enough to revive the energetic system so MMT can begin. The wonderful thing about FBA is it allows the practitioner to test anything she feels may be beneficial or harmful to a patient's health. When all goes well, the doctor can simply place a substance on or very near the body and evaluate the response through a test-muscle. As explained thoroughly in the chapter, *Functional Bio-Analysis: What, How, Why*, the body constantly monitors and evaluates electromagnetic fields—the energetic fingerprint manifested by all things. It does so without ceasing, just like it does with smells, touch and any of the five physical senses.

The problem is any sample substance that generates a field is naturally quite weak. This is similar to a radio broadcast. If the receiver is out of range, or if things like mountains, tunnels or power lines interrupt the signal, the music will not be properly heard. The stresses of life, be they chemical, structural or emotional, are mountains of an electromagnetic sort. Medications, toxins or other stresses act like foreign frequencies and activate the survival response or distort the incoming electromagnetic transmissions. In order for FBA to be reliable, the practitioner needs to tune the body so that the patient's body can "hear" the electromagnetic broadcast of the tested substances.

Additionally, practitioners can aid the body's detection of frequencies by enhancing or boosting the signal of the substance being tested. By using a magnet and placing a substance under the south-pole side or by using a source of light (sunlight is the best), practitioners can boost the signal. Both of these techniques add energy to the equation and intensify the signal making it easier for the body to detect the fingerprint.

In order to know whether the body is ready for FBA, the practitioner can utilize a very special reflex point on the top of the head called Governing Vessel 20 (GV20). Touching that point should weaken a test-muscle. This rarely happens when a patient first lies down on the treatment table. Once GV 20 is open (weakens to a test-muscle), the body has removed enough current stress and is relaxed. The patient is now ready for Functional Bio-Analysis.

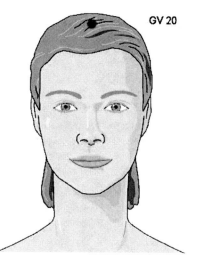

GV 20

PRIMARY ENERGETIC POINTS – WHAT TO FIX FIRST?

According to traditional acupuncture, energetic points literally cover the human body from head to toe. FBA takes into consideration 15 of these points, called primary energetic points (PEPs). Each corresponds with an organ or system of the body. In addition, 14 of the 15 points relate to high or low levels of seven special hormones called neurotransmitters, which perform critical functions in the brain and elsewhere. The chapters that follow are based on the major symptoms related to each primary reflex point and its corresponding neurotransmitter. For example, the chapter, *Pleasure or Paranoia?* is related to the PEP governing vessel 27 (GV27) and has to do with high levels of the neurotransmitter dopamine. The chapter *Panic or Pass Out?* describes the symptoms related to an excess of the excitatory neurotransmitter norepinephrine, which discovered through the PEP, Heart 1 (HRT 1).

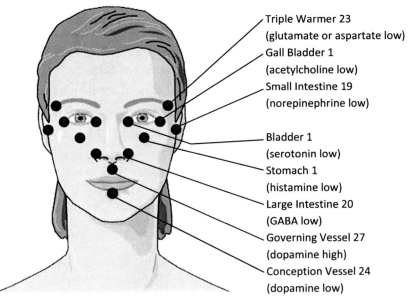

Triple Warmer 23
(glutamate or aspartate low)
Gall Bladder 1
(acetylcholine low)
Small Intestine 19
(norepinephrine low)

Bladder 1
(serotonin low)
Stomach 1
(histamine low)
Large Intestine 20
(GABA low)
Governing Vessel 27
(dopamine high)
Conception Vessel 24
(dopamine low)

Figure 6: Facial PEPs - Low Neurotransmitters

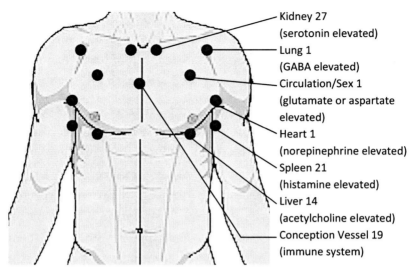

Figure 7: Body PEPs - High Neurotransmitters

With a gentle touch of the reflex point and the response of a test-muscle, a practitioner can quickly determine whether a given neurotransmitter is high, low, or balanced. To correct the ones out of balance, he can make use of the hormetic nutrients associated with each reflex point.

It is not a coincidence that the most important reflex points on the body correlate with neurotransmitters. Neurophysiology is an advancing field of study and practice based upon the idea that most problems start in the brain and work their way down. By making treatment of brain dysfunction a priority, chiropractic neurologists have used specific manual therapies to do amazing things - helping patients in ways traditional methods could not. This is exactly what happens with FBA but from a chemical point of view. By fixing the neurotransmitters found through the primary reflex points, the practitioner can manage the patient's highest priorities from a top-down perspective while correcting both the brain and the body at the same time.

Once the primary energetic point (PEP) is found, a basic thought process for the practitioner begins as he puts to use his biochemical understanding in order to discern the most appropriate treatment. The ideas regarding neurotransmitters and hormones are foundational for all of the PEP chapters that follow.

NAVIGATING THE PATHWAYS

In order for FBA practitioners to be effective, they must understand certain aspects of biochemistry. Specifically, how the body makes, or synthesizes, a neurotransmitter or hormone and then breaks it down, or metabolizes it. After making or obtaining biochemical substances, the body must utilize them, get rid of them, or recycle them. A failure within any of these basic steps means a functional problem will be present. Simply put, restoring health often comes down to balancing a hormone or neurotransmitter that is either too high or too low. An excess or deficiency will cause remarkable symptoms, and the PEP corresponding to the out-of-balance substance will become active. This means the issue is now detectable with manual muscle testing.

To understand how the body builds neurotransmitters and metabolic chemicals, think of Legos, a favorite toy of all children. Using Legos, a child may build a bus, turn it into a car, and then make it into a plane—all with the appropriate rearrangement and addition or subtraction of only a few other pieces. The body builds neurotransmitters in much the same way. There is very little chemical difference, for example, between dopamine and adrenaline, yet they have unrelated functions. Understanding how these "blocks" connect together and what they need to transform into their next shape is an important way to determine whether there is a problem.

Another way to think about hormones and neurotransmitters is to imagine their normal pathway as a steady flowing river passing by several towns making use of the water. If each upstream town only draws what it needs, then plenty of water is available for the remaining towns downstream. However, abuse, droughts, and dams disperse the water unevenly.

To better understand the point, compare the two pathways for the neurotransmitter serotonin below.

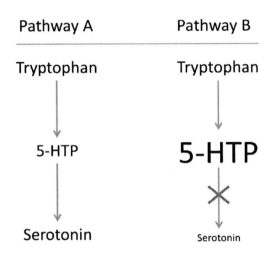

Figure 8: Serotonin Pathway

To make serotonin, the body begins with an amino acid called tryptophan. Once used, it is reshaped into 5-HTP and then finally into serotonin. Pathway A is an example of a river properly flowing from one "neuro-town" to the next, each town using just the amount of water it needs. Pathway B has a big problem. Just below the town of 5-HTP there is a blockage. Apparently, some beavers have decided to build a dam in this spot. Now, Sero-town is drying up. The result is an excess of 5-HTP and a deficiency of serotonin.

Excesses of neurotransmitters mean water will eventually overflow the banks, making a messy bug-breeding pond. Deficiencies, on the other hand are like a drought; there will not be enough water for the crops or the animals and people to drink. Both of these situations are unhealthy. Each PEP has a pathway and requires certain hormetic nutrients to keep it flowing. Finding the areas where the neurotransmitters are dammed up and helping remove the blockage is a powerful way to encourage health.

A common approach to regulate low neurotransmitters is simply to supplement with an "upstream" substance or substrate like tryptophan or

5-HTP. This approach only works in the case where the substrate itself is low. Otherwise, when a blockage is present, adding additional substrate will result in no improvement or worse yet, may yield unexpected side effects. Therefore, it becomes imperative for the practitioner to know the condition of each substrate, determine whether it is in disarray, and repair it accordingly.

Once a pathway seems balanced by the hormetic nutrients, there are two things practitioners should consider to assist with long-term healing and to make sure the same problem does not come back. First, it is always good to put as much stress on the pathway as possible, to "flood the river," and see whether the hormetic nutrients can still keep the PEP balanced. Second, based on the Teeter-Totter Effect, if one neurotransmitter or hormone is too high, another is probably too low. In the case of serotonin, once its pathway seems solid, it would be a good idea to check the PEPs for high and low dopamine.

Flooding the River

Any issue of a chronic nature has layers that can run deep. Managing the superficial layers, as well as tapping into and correcting the deeper hidden ones, is essential for a complete recovery. Likewise, health-related problems can come and go. Doctors often hear their patients say things like, "Well, my back hurt yesterday when I called for this appointment, but today it seems just fine." By recreating the "real world" where patients actually live, practitioners can find hidden structural problems. For instance, a doctor may stress a patient's tissues by having them move, bend, or run in place. Introducing any form of stress and evaluating the body's response, is likely to provide beneficial insight. For example, a hormetic nutrient may cancel the muscle weakness from a PEP, but will it continue to do so under stress? One quick way to find out is by placing a patient's genetic color over their eyes. Genetic colors are a form of energetic stress. Now, the practitioner can retest to see if it the nutrient still prevents a muscle from weakening to the PEP. If so, it demonstrates that this particular hormetic nutrient will continue to provide a therapeutic response even in the midst of additional strain.

Other times, instead of finding the most effective nutrient to retain physiologic integrity, the goal is to see what substances cause a pathway to breakdown. Intentionally overwhelming a pathway reveals potential areas of weakness. The most common stress or "challenge" to the metabolic pathways is with particular chemicals called biomarkers.

SPEED UP THE PROCESS WITH BIOMARKERS

Biomarkers are the substances most directly related to a given PEP. Using biomarkers tells the FBA practitioner exactly what is wrong with the PEP and is the fastest way to find the most appropriate hormetic nutrient to fix it. With any PEP, there could be up to 10 hormetic nutrients to check in order to find the one that works best. Biomarkers narrow down the search to just one or two hormetic nutrients. For example, if SPL 21 is active, then the FBA practitioner knows a problem with the blood sugar system is present. He could check all the hormetic nutrients related to this PEP and thereby fix the problem. But he would not know why the problem was there in the first place. Only the biomarker can tell him that. The good news is the hormetic nutrient that brings the biomarker into balance tends also to be the one bringing the entire PEP into balance. In the case of SPL 21, the biomarkers are glycogen, insulin, glucose, and glucagon. Using FBA, a practitioner can test small samples of these substances to see whether a strong test-muscle becomes weak.

Using a biomarker not only leads the practitioner to the problem, but it also reveals precisely what kind of problem is present. If glycogen happened to be the biomarker that stabilized SPL 21, it would instantly narrow down the possibilities for hormetic nutrients to just three things: cortisol, calcium, and vitamin B6. Cortisol and calcium help make glycogen, and vitamin B6 helps release it from storage when the body needs it.

PEP Summary

The primary energetic points of FBA all relate to 15 major bodily systems and their specific pathways and chemicals. All these systems, with the exception of one, have an association with hormones or neurotransmitters - the hormones of the brain. This relationship means that with the gentle touch of the reflex point and the response of a test-muscle, an FBA practitioner can quickly determine whether a given neurotransmitter is high, low, or balanced. Therefore, balancing PEPs requires an understanding of the major biochemical pathways.

To correct the ones out of balance, he can make use of the hormetic nutrients associated with each reflex point. Certain special chemicals associated with these pathways called biomarkers are substances directly related to a PEP, and an FBA practitioner can use them to speed up the overall evaluative process. This makes finding the necessary hormetic nutrient much easier. By definition, hormetic nutrients are involved in numerous essential pathways. One may well seem helpful initially but turn out not to be the best choice overall. To ensure a practitioner has found the most effective hormetic nutrient to balance the PEP, he may need to add structural, chemical, emotional, or even energetic stresses to see whether the PEP will still maintain its integrity. If the PEP is unable to resist additional stresses, the practitioner should look for another hormetic nutrient to making the PEP stable under additional stress. Lastly, certain special circumstances related to hormones and how they behave in the body need consideration, lest the full restoration of PEPs be prevented.

HYPOGLYCEMIA OR HISTAMINE? – SPLEEN 21

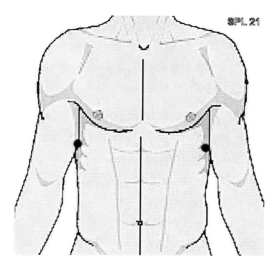

Figure 9: Spleen 21

Related Neurotransmitter: Histamine (high levels)

Organ or System: Spleen & Blood Sugar System

Main Biomarkers: Insulin, Glycogen, Glucose, Cortisol, Histamine

Common Hormetic Nutrients: B6, Calcium, Thiamin (B1), Alpha-Lipoic Acid, B12, Vanadium, Chromium

Spleen 21 (SP 21) is located on both sides of the rib cage, about four inches below the armpit. It is the PEP related to the spleen and, perhaps more importantly, the pancreas, which is the manufacturing plant for insulin. As a hormone, insulin is critical for proper blood sugar balance. Of the fifteen primary energetic points discussed in *Hope for Health*, many practitioners consider SP 21 to be the most important for overcoming functional illness. The reason is simple. SP 21 has everything to do with managing blood sugar, or glucose, and glucose is the main fuel for the brain. Therefore, in order to keep the brain supplied with ample amounts of fuel, the body places SP 21 at the top of its priority list and makes whatever sacrifices are necessary to keep this system up and running. Beyond this, glucose relates to all functions of the body because every cell needs it for fuel. It is not just brain fuel; it is body fuel as well. As a practitioner uses FBA to reveal the priorities of the body, it is likely he will find SP 21 among the top three primary energetic points, no matter what the type of functional illness.

The blood sugar system intimately connects with the adrenal glands, thyroid glands, and reproductive system. Strain on any one of these places will bring about strain on the rest. Like a debt-based government protecting entities too big to fail, the blood sugar system, when desperate, will borrow whatever resources it can from its dependent partners, exhausting them and eventually itself. This undesirable outcome is most often the result of poor choices. The Western diet, full of processed oils, refined foods, and plenty of sweeteners, along with inadequate sleep and the worries of life are the principal trouble-makers. Although, a bad diet is enough stress on its own.

Even with plenty of sleep and few worries, children often experience significant blood sugar stress from the food they eat. The rise in juvenile or Type 1 diabetes should give parents pause. Each year, physicians diagnose more than 15,000 children and teenagers with type 1 diabetes in the U.S.[239] In some countries, like Finland and Australia, the rates are much worse.[240]

METABOLIC SYNDROME

Today, the Western world is suffering from a myriad of individual metabolic disorders that, as a group, have the name Metabolic Syndrome.[241] At its core, Metabolic Syndrome is a blood sugar problem. Those with Metabolic Syndrome who are also obese carry yet another label: Syndrome X. Current estimates from the American Heart Association report that 20-25 percent of the adult population of the U.S. suffers from Syndrome X. This means between 58 and 73 million men and women are at risk for this disorder. Many more are at risk from Metabolic Syndrome, because they are not classified as obese but have all the other associated aliments.

Metabolic Syndrome is characterized by having at least three of the following symptoms:

- Insulin Resistance (high insulin and high blood sugar)
- Abdominal fat—in men this means a 40-inch waist or larger, in women 35 inches or larger
- High blood sugar levels—at least 110 mg/dl after fasting
- Triglycerides elevated—at least 150 mg/dl in the blood stream
- Low HDL (the "good" cholesterol)—less than 40 mg/dl if male and 50 mg/dl if female
- A tendency to clot, called a prothrombotic state
- Blood pressure of 130/85 or higher

If present, Metabolic Syndrome greatly increases the chances of having a heart attack or stroke. The medical community understands these illnesses "cluster" together. Meaning they connect to each other through a vicious cycle where one condition perpetuates the prevalence and severity of another. Despite knowing this, the American Heart Association, a group of traditional medical doctors, states on its website that the "underlying causes of Metabolic Syndrome are being overweight, physical inactivity, and genetic factors."[242] These are causes? They are not causes; they are signs and symptoms.

In those with Metabolic Syndrome, the fuse was lit well before the bomb went off. The metabolic causes were present for decades. Failure to understand the basic mechanisms of the blood sugar system and its interactions with the rest of the hormonal system leaves little hope for patients under the care of traditional doctors. This is why the best traditional medicine can offer is condition-management through medications and why it rarely finds cures or prevents anything. So, what are the real causes of metabolic syndrome and all other functional blood sugar disorders?

The Glucose Pathway

In order to benefit from glucose, the body must follow and maintain hundreds of steps while meeting specific conditions. A simplified version of the glucose pathway could be expressed something like this: glucose must be obtained through digestion, transported to the cell via insulin, overseen by cortisol (an adrenal gland hormone), received into the cell by trace minerals, utilized in the cell's mitochondria, stored as glycogen in the liver and muscles, retrieved when needed by a hormone called glucagon, and finally, when not needed, stored as fat. If trouble is present anywhere in the glucose pathway, there is a functional problem. Within these steps is *the cause* of Metabolic Syndrome and of many other functional illnesses. It is essential therefore, that these potential problem areas be examined.

Rarely will a patient ever express to his doctor all the ailments he is currently suffering from. If done so, the five-minute visit to the HMO physician would likely result in a prescription for an anti-depressant. This is no joke. When asked, most people are managing symptoms of pain, insomnia, digestive complains, hormonal issues, headaches, and fatigue. Far too often, people function daily by forcing metabolic reactions to take place. "I need my morning coffee," they grumble. The 2:30 crash amidst a monstrous sugar craving is no concern since a bowl of chocolate candies on Sally's desk is easily within reach. These symptoms all directly relate to a struggling blood sugar system and lead from health to functional illness and from functional illness to disease.

Insulin & Glycogen

The human body stores fuel in three forms: lipids in the fat tissue; proteins as muscle; and sugars, called glycogen. Three hormones (glucagon, cortisol, and norepinephrine) increase blood sugar levels, but only one, namely insulin, gets blood sugar into the cells. In other words, the body is three times better able to manage food shortages than it is food excesses. This biological fact is the reason why those with lowered caloric intake have some of the greatest longevity. Centenarians, those living to 100 years old or more, no matter their gender, race, or location in the world, have two things in common. They never over eat, they are free from autoimmune attack, and they maintain a happy or positive attitude.[243] [244] In civilized society, with its abundant options of quick and easy grease- and sweet-filled foods, keeping calories down could be one of life's greatest challenges.

Insulin is a hormone made by the pancreas in response to the presence of glucose in the blood stream, usually following a meal. It is the job of insulin to shepherd glucose into a cell so the cell can use it as fuel. When performing properly, blood sugar levels will be within an optimal fasting range of 85-100 mg/dl. If the cells are no longer responding to insulin as they should, then blood sugar levels will tend to dramatically move above and below the range. Many practitioners consider high blood sugar to be a "silent" disease. It often has few symptoms initially. On the other hand doctors recognize low blood sugar, called hypoglycemia, by symptoms between meals, such as irritability, lightheadedness, sugar cravings, sleeplessness at night, memory loss, fatigue, and more.

In the muscles, liver, and kidneys, an 8- to 10-hour supply of stored glucose, called glycogen, is available.[245] The presence of a functional calcium deficiency, especially the kind that happens in BLUE people, can hinder glycogen production. Low cortisol levels can also contribute to a problem in glycogen production. Cortisol, a hormone produced by the outer part, or cortex of the adrenal glands, will be insufficient in those who have chronic stress. People with chronic stress fatigue the glands, and they are no longer able to meet demand. There is also a second problem. Glycogen can become stuck in storage. The key that unlocks the glycogen cabinet is vitamin B6, or pyridoxine.[246] B6 is an important hormetic nutrient and, for many reasons, is a common nutrient deficiency. Inability to create or access glycogen is the main reason for civilized society's epidemic of hypoglycemia.

HYPOGLYCEMIA

Hypoglycemics are people who experience low levels of glucose in their blood stream. Typical symptoms include: craving sweets, lightheadedness, shakiness, low energy, and headaches. All these occur between meals. Because the body works so hard to maintain stable blood sugar levels and sacrifices other systems when necessary by stealing their required nutrients, a person whose glucose levels are not within normal ranges already has a serious metabolic imbalance underway. For example, hypoglycemics generally have plenty of stored fuel in the form of fat but are no longer able to use their foundational energy reserve. This, as explained below, is the result of the fight-or-flight response and is the reason why many hypoglycemics cannot lose weight even with a yeoman's effort. Other signs are also present when the blood sugar system is strained. In fact, because of its influence over so many bodily systems, any blood sugar problem means that a cluster of functional issues are present simultaneously.

Hypoglycemics are not usually hungry in the morning. That is because they have been under stress all night. Imagine Cynthia on her way to meet friends for a late dinner at a popular restaurant. One block before she arrives, a mother pushing her baby in a stroller walks directly out in front of the car. Luckily, Cynthia sees them in time, slams the brakes, and averts tragedy. However, inside her body everything has changed. The mild hunger pangs and the pleasant thoughts of her favorite meal are now gone. A surge of adrenaline has activated the sympathetic nervous system. Her heart is racing, her pupils are dilated, and her breathing is rapid and shallow. Blood flow is also diverted away from the digestive organs and into the big muscles. Cynthia is experiencing a full-blown fight-or-flight response. The process, once begun, takes time to diminish. With her appetite gone, Cynthia retells the event to her friends while occasionally sipping on some wine. After an hour, she is finally able to have a few bites of her favorite course but is still trembling on the inside. This illustration is a dramatic example of what happens every night in the body of the hypoglycemic.

Only a few hours after dinner, as hypoglycemics curl up in bed to go to sleep, glucose levels begin to drop. With no food in sight, their bodies must find some blood sugar in order to fuel the brain. The glycogen cabinets in the liver and kidneys are either empty or locked. In either case, the normal means of acquiring glucose are not options. So, the body takes an emergency measure. It releases adrenaline, one of the chief fight-or-flight hormones, in order to make glucose from the muscles, a process called gluconeogenesis. Prolonged destruction of muscle for fuel is a highly inflammatory and nutrient-depleting process, worsening an already serious functional problem and creating restless sleep.

All night long, the hypoglycemic tosses and turns as his body tries to find rest in a state of high sympathetic activity. Getting up to go to the bathroom for the second time, he reminds himself not to drink water before bed. This has little to do with the problem. Night time urination is rarely an issue when the blood sugar system is properly working. The chemicals from the fight-or-flight response are toxic, and the body must eliminate the toxins through the kidneys as soon as possible, even at the expense of sleep. This is why night-time urination in the hypoglycemic is unavoidable. When sleep does occur, vivid dreams, the result of an overactive liver processing the same noxious chemicals as the kidneys, often keep it from being restful. When morning finally arrives, the fight-or-flight response has been at work for many hours, and so appetite, like in Cynthia's case above, is absent.

Even though hypoglycemics have little desire for breakfast, skipping the morning meal is one of the worst things they can do. It allows for the further perpetuation of the body's muscle-stripping emergency measures in order to retrieve glucose. Instead, forcing the body to move in a different direction by changing lifestyle habits is essential. This means eating a protein-based meal even if a person can only tolerate a few bites. Usually, half a hardboiled egg with a piece of toast and a bite of a green vegetable is sufficient. This dietary step is critical because the degenerative disorders linked to high ingestion of refined carbohydrates are many, including the following ones: [247]

- Arthritis
- Autoimmune Disorders
- Cancer
- Chronic Fatigue
- Diabetes
- Fibromyalgia
- Heart Disease
- Hypo and hyperthyroidism.

Since the mid 1990's, books, such as *The Adkin's Diet, The Zone, The Paleo Diet, Protein Power*, and the *South Beach Diet* have recommended controlling blood sugar levels by eating higher amounts of protein. Each of these books works to correct the glucose imbalances the fight-or-flight response and the over-consumption of refined foods and sugars create. These diets are not without their problems. Too much protein has concerns of its own. However, if they help people overcome their addiction to sugar while balancing their blood sugar system at the same time, they will have done a great service to the population as a whole.

Remember, blood sugar problems are part of most functional illnesses. Without their correction, the body cannot fix certain significant illnesses. To make matters worse, prolonged hypoglycemia leads to even more serious blood sugar problems, such as insulin resistance and diabetes.

Correcting Hypoglycemia with FBA

There are four main substances to consider when evaluating hypoglycemia: insulin, glycogen, glucose, and glucagon. Samples of these substances, called biomarkers, are evaluated by the FBA practitioner through manual muscle testing.

The chart shows the three primary blood sugar imbalances—hypoglycemia, insulin resistance, and diabetes—and the relationship of the four main biomarkers, whether they are too high, too low, or normal. Testing the biomarkers with FBA will reveal a patient's current blood sugar category.

Condition	Glucose	Insulin	Glycogen	Cortisol
Hypoglycemia	↓	↑ or normal	↓ or ↑	↑ then ↓
Insulin Resistance	↑	↑	↓ or ↑	↑ then ↓
Diabetes	↑	↓	↓	↓

In the case of hypoglycemia, the answer is almost always glycogen. As in the chart above, glycogen will either be high or low. This is because the body either has a manufacturing problem and consequently glycogen output is low, or the body already has plenty of glycogen but needs to make better use of what it already has. The more common of these two problems is low levels of glycogen. To make this important glucose-storing molecule, the body requires plenty of usable calcium and a hormone from the adrenal glands called cortisol.

Since glycogen is something the body would like to have, simply placing a sample of it on the body temporarily excites the nervous system. This facilitating response is enough to cause a weak test-muscle to become strong. Next, the practitioner can check for calcium in its various forms and/or cortisol. One of the two will also excite the nervous system. When one does, the practitioner has found a large piece of the hypoglycemia puzzle. The person should take the needed nutrient in supplement form while correcting lifestyle choices contributing to the problem. For some, just one of these two nutrients is sufficient. For others, the metabolic issues are far more complex.

A second problem that can cause hypoglycemia has to do with the inefficient use of glycogen. There is plenty of it in the storage cabinets, but the cabinets are locked and no one can find the key. When glycogen is stuck in storage, the key that lets it out is vitamin B6, called pyridoxine. In some cases (usually cases involving genetic issues) only the activated form of B6 will do. Most activated forms of vitamins have a phosphorous molecule attached to them. Thus pyridoxine in its activated form would be called pyridoxal-5-phosphate. People with this particular low-glucose problem have plenty of calcium and cortisol from their adrenal glands but have somewhere along the way been stripped of B-vitamins. B6 is more than just a key for glycogen cabinets. In the nervous system it is used to relax tingling and trapped nerves;[248] in the brain it helps process neurotransmitters and aids in seizure reduction;[249] in the mitochondria, it helps promote energy creation; and in the spleen, it is essential to metabolize histamine, the chemical found in high amounts during allergic reactions.

A final form of hypoglycemia has to do with the inability of the cells themselves to absorb glucose. This occurs when there is a shortage of either chromium or vanadium—the doorman and the butler. It is the job of insulin to escort glucose to the cell. Once it arrives, insulin knocks on the cell door and waits for the doorman. The doorman is chromium.[250] Without this important trace mineral, the door stays closed. In other words, there could be plenty of glucose available for energy but if it can't get into the cell, it is for all practical purposes useless. If the doorman does open the door, the body needs to take another step. The butler must welcome glucose into the cellular mansion. The butler is vanadium, another important trace mineral. A quick check of these biomarkers with FBA will ensure the body is making and releasing glycogen, and that glucose will be able to get into, and be used by, the cells.

INSULIN RESISTANCE

Insulin resistance is the condition in which normal amounts of insulin are inadequate to produce normal responses.[251] Therefore, the pancreas must produce higher levels. This is a dangerous place to be. The pancreas can only deliver high levels of insulin for a period of time before petering out. The end result is diabetes. This process does not happen overnight, but it is the consequence of longstanding blood sugar stress.

Insulin resistance prevents the efficient conversion of food into energy because of a vastly reduced number of insulin receptors on the cell wall. Doctors estimate that a typical healthy person has 20,000 insulin receptor sites per cell, while the average overweight individual can have as few as 5,000. This phenomenon directly relates to high carbohydrate consumption, which results in bountiful amounts of glucose in the blood stream. This too is very dangerous. Excess glucose can bind with and alter proteins resulting in what are called advanced glycosylated end products (AGE's). These substances increase arteriosclerosis and rapidly advance the aging process.[252]

Continuous exposure to anything can result in a desensitizing effect. This is true even for cells bombarded with glucose. The body finds some way to deal with the excessive stimulation at first. Since the cellular house is already full of glucose-guests, it cannot allow any more in. So it does the next best thing and turns a deaf ear. As insulin continues knocking at the door, the doorman refuses to answer. The over-stimulation has desensitized the cell to the presence of insulin. The only response the body has is to send out more knockers. This extreme measure, in time, will take its toll on the pancreas. To make matters worse, excess or free-floating insulin is dangerous. For example, too much insulin is highly inflammatory and can damage the lining of the arteries and contribute to the development of atherosclerosis.

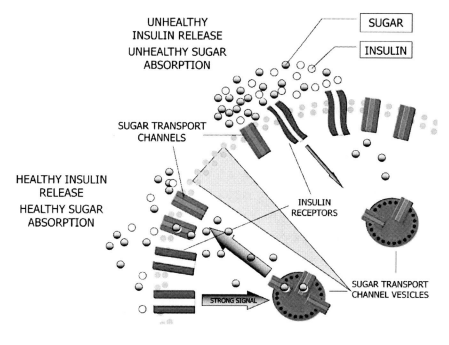

Figure 10: Insulin Resistance

Insulin has influence over more than just glucose. Fat, muscle, and liver cells must also respond to insulin's call. In the presence of insulin resistance, blood levels of triglycerides, free fatty acids, and, of course, blood sugar will rise.[253] Remember, high blood levels of insulin and glucose combined are a marker for Metabolic Syndrome, as well as type 2 diabetes.[254] Research has indicated increased insulin and glucose levels cause changes in the kidneys' ability to remove salt, as well as increasing the risk of blood clot formation.[255] All these are key factors in the development of cardiovascular disease, heart attacks, and stroke.[256] It should now be clear why blood sugar issues are the thread that unravels the sweater of Metabolic Syndrome and many other functional illnesses, as well.

Correcting Insulin Resistance with FBA

The biomarker for insulin resistance is insulin itself. When the practitioner exposes the patient to this compound and a test-muscle weakens, it indicates the body already has plenty of insulin and that insulin is now causing harm. Therefore, insulin resistance is likely. Getting this situation under control requires hormetic nutrients. The most common ones are the activated form of vitamin B1 called, thiamin pyrophosphate, followed by alpha lipoic acid and/or a specific form of vitamin B12. Just like there can be genetic issues activating vitamin B6 in certain patients when glycogen is stuck in storage, there is often a genetic problem activating vitamin B1 with insulin resistance. Thiamin inactivation has ramifications for many other conditions, including scoliosis, a deforming condition of the spine.

With insulin still on the body, the practitioner can check the hormetic nutrients to see whether the inhibition abates and strength returns. Usually, only one of these hormetic nutrients will work. The person should take the one that works in supplement form as part of her nutritional schedule. Since the glucose pathway is multifaceted, checking for other blood sugars issues is critical for maximum therapeutic results. A practitioner can do this simply by leaving the balancing hormetic nutrient on the body and then checking other biomarkers to see whether they need balancing, as well. Again, lifestyle changes, such as specialized diets and exercise routines, are critical to support and reinforce the nutritional therapies.

HISTAMINE

SPL 21, as the name suggests, relates to the spleen. The spleen has everything to do with the management of a chemical called histamine. High levels of histamine will activate SPL 21, which is then detectable with FBA. The effects of histamine are quite familiar. Watery eyes, itchy nose, sneezing, and scratching are all common in the presence of allergic reactions triggered by histamine. Histamine is also a neurotransmitter in the brain synthesized from an amino acid called histidine.

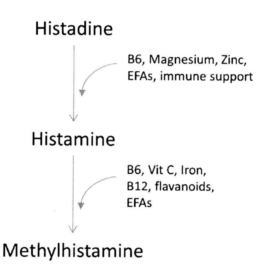

Figure 11: Histamine Pathway

The pathway above shows the synthesis and metabolism of histamine and the nutrients required to make those steps happen. If a biomarker of histamine creates a weakness in a strong test-muscle, then too much of this noxious chemical is circulating in the body. A hormetic nutrient of vitamin B6, iron, or vitamin C is necessary to help reduce histamine levels.

Allergies related to histamine are not always this easy to fix. This occurs because histamine is part of other pathways not shown above, each of which requires a different hormetic nutrient. The greater the number of imbalanced pathways, the more difficult it can be to fix a given problem. This is why fixing allergies is sometimes tricky and why over-the-counter medications may work for some people and do nothing for others. The good news is that the experienced FBA practitioner is aware of these other pathways and can quickly check for and find the appropriate hormetic nutrient(s).

SAD OR SLEEPLESS? – BLADDER 1

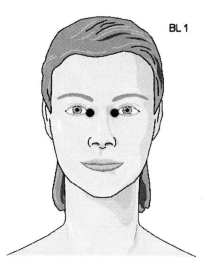

Figure 12: Bladder 1

Related Neurotransmitter: Serotonin (low levels)

Organ or System: Bladder

Main Biomarkers: L-Tryptophan, Serotonin, Melatonin

Common Hormetic Nutrients: Magnesium, B6, Zinc, Calcium, B12

Insomnia and depression are two of the most common complaints among those visiting a doctor.[257] Both directly relate to the PEP, Bladder 1 (BL 1), which is located deep in the inner corner of the eyes. The bladder energy meridian in acupuncture is one of the most important for doctors of Chinese medicine because of its influence over all meridians of the body. Along with SPL 1, BL 1 is often a top three PEP when evaluated with FBA. The biochemical pathway associated with this point contains three elements that many people have already heard of: tryptophan, serotonin and melatonin. Tryptophan is the "sleepy" amino acid found in turkey meat, serotonin is the neurotransmitter that keeps people happy (or at least not depressed), and melatonin is the critical hormone for deep sleep. Here is what the pathway looks like:

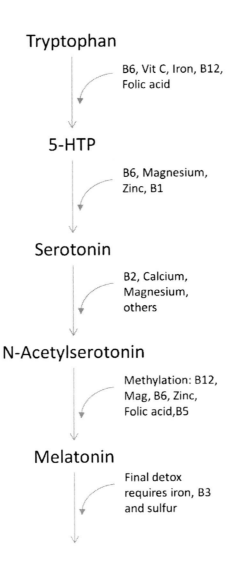

Figure 13: The Serotonin Pathway

When BL 1 is positive, bringing it back into balance it means evaluating the three main biomarkers (tryptophan, serotonin, and melatonin) with FBA. In order for this pathway to begin flowing, plenty of tryptophan, an *essential* amino acid, must be present. Chemical substances in the body are either essential or non-essential. If a substance is essential, it means the body must obtain it from the diet. If a substance is non-essential, it means that the body can synthesize it from other elements already present. Tryptophan must be obtained from food. The benefits of this amino acid for sleep, anxiety reduction, mood stability and neuropsychiatric disorders are well known.[258] The reason it works is because it floods the happy-mood-and-sleep pathway with plenty of raw material to make serotonin and melatonin. However, this assumes the pathway is free from obstruction.

If tryptophan is effective for someone, then the logical question is: why did he or she need more of it in the first place? There are three reasons why tryptophan may be low:

1. *A low protein diet* – Since amino acids are the building blocks of protein, and tryptophan is an amino acid, tryptophan levels will be low if there is not enough protein.

2. *Poor digestion* – All the protein in the world won't help a person if the body lacks the ability to properly process it into its most basic parts - amino acids. Digesting protein requires adequate stomach acid. Prolonged emotional stress often leads to low hydrochloric acid production in the stomach and consequently low protein digestion. If protein digestion is properly begun in the stomach, there could still be trouble further down the tract. Full and complete digestion takes place in a healthy small intestine. However, if this tissue becomes inflamed from too many processed foods or perhaps as the result of an infection, it becomes leaky, a phenomenon called, Leaky Gut Syndrome (LGS). When present, LGS prevents full digestion of proteins, and the body will not be able to harvest sufficient amounts of tryptophan.

3. *The Liver Thief* – Believe it or not, there are more important things to the body than how a person feels. Keeping an individual alive is one of them. Fungal or yeast overgrowth in the digestive tract, or elsewhere, is a serious matter. The waste products of these unwanted critters are extremely toxic, and the liver devotes an entire pathway to breaking down these noxious substances. But, there is a catch. Tryptophan is the main detoxifying agent. Therefore, when necessary, the liver will steal tryptophan meant for the brain in order to keep the body from becoming overly polluted, which is a much worse state.

The FBA practitioner must consider each of these possibilities whenever a patient shows a need for tryptophan. More often, however, the problem is not too little tryptophan but a failure to breakdown what is already there. In this case, patient-exposure to tryptophan will cause a strong test muscle to become weak. Finding the hormetic nutrient to fix this issue is the answer.

DEPRESSION – LOW SEROTONIN

Neurotransmitters are the hormones of the brain. They are responsible for how we relate, remember and react to the world around us. Symptoms of serotonin irregularities are commonplace and include the following ones:

- Depression
- Lacking artistic expression
- Loss of enjoyment for favorite foods and hobbies
- Lower pain tolerance
- Dependency on others
- Disrupted sleep
- Feelings of paranoia

Serotonin is perhaps the most recognized neurotransmitter. The reason for this awareness is simply because serotonin is the main neurotransmitter related to depression. The cost of depression and other mental illnesses is nearly 300 billion dollars annually. Over seven million women in the United States have clinical depression, according to the National Mental Health Association. Women are twice as likely as men to suffer from depression, indicating a strong hormonal connection to the problem.

About 10 percent of Americans, or 30 million people, are currently taking anti-depressants. That number is double what it was only a decade earlier and has shown no signs of slowing down.[259] [260]

The type of medication most taken for depression is an SSRI, or a selective serotonin reuptake inhibitor. It is the job of these medications to prevent the body from processing serotonin. The result is people feel better. This sounds good, but it is not without significant problems. Re-uptake prevention will insure plenty of serotonin remains in the brain but leaves the downstream substances, like melatonin, in a drought. This perhaps is why so many people taking anti-depressants also need to take sleep aids at the same time. Remember, serotonin is but one step in a sophisticated and somewhat fragile pathway. The goal of FBA is to fix the broken pathways, not to simply support a single member.

Anti-depressants have a few dark secrets, as well. Prolonged or even shorter use of anti-depressants can suppress immune function,[261] [262] effect sexual function[263] and may even promote suicide.[264] The overall effectiveness of SSRIs is also coming under scrutiny. Scientists at Duke University Medical Center tested exercise against the drug Zoloft and found the ability of either, or a combination of the two, to reduced or eliminated symptoms was about the same percentage. However, they found exercise seemed to do a better job of keeping symptoms from coming back after the depression lifted. Their findings, reported in the *Journal of Psychosomatic Medicine*, suggest a modest exercise program "is an effective, robust treatment for patients with major depression."[265] Simply put, SSRIs do not and cannot fix broken pathways.

There is a close connection between stress levels and depression. Second only to blood sugar imbalances, the serotonin pathway may be the most susceptible to damage from the effects of emotional stress.[266] [267] In the modern world, reducing stress must be intentional. For the sake of health, a person should consider lifestyle choices, career paths, peripheral relationships and commitments of all types based upon the potential increases in emotional and physical stress. The new "busy" is far too busy for the body, which has limits. Too much ongoing stress drains the hormetic nutrients necessary to synthesize serotonin and all other neurotransmitters. High levels of serotonin are in no way good either. They are a trigger for migraine headaches. As expected, since migraines are such a severe issue, the body should have a way through the energetic points to warn us, and it does. See the chapter, *Migraines, Metals, or Minerals* for the details.

From a neurological point of view, depression results from low firing of the frontal cortex. Brain stimulation in the form of new challenges and body movement is also important. See the *Brain Rehab* section in the chapter, *ADHD or Misplaced Memory?*, for some helpful suggestions.

INSOMNIA & MELATONIN

Melatonin is the fifth substance in the serotonin pathway and is one of the most important chemicals for deep sleep. Almost all people with functional illnesses suffer from one or more forms of insomnia. As a health problem, insomnia is a widespread issue. A general consensus, developed from population-based studies, reports that approximately 30 percent of adults from different countries experience one or more of the symptoms of insomnia: difficulty initiating sleep; difficulty maintaining sleep; waking up too early; and in some cases, nonrestorative or poor quality of sleep.[268] These folks are heading for trouble. Melatonin is cancer protective;[269] [270] aids the immune system in infection, inflammation and autoimmunity;[271] [272] and may help keep a person young.[273] Promoting melatonin production through a healthy sleep cycle is a must for health.

Adequate melatonin levels depend upon plenty of light during the day and plenty of dark at night. Direct daily sunlight is critical for normal circadian rhythms and to stimulate the pineal gland, which is the gland in the brain responsible for increasing melatonin levels when it is dark.[274] Usually 15 to 30 minutes of sunlight is enough. Artificial light in the nighttime hours, however, has a strong negative impact on melatonin production. Night shift work, staying up late viewing the television or the computer, or just keeping things bright up until bedtime will all decrease melatonin levels.[275]

When a person has insomnia, he or she will often take melatonin in supplement form. This should only be done for a period less than eight or ten weeks so as not to develop a dependency on this hormone. However, only a small percentage of people will benefit from this approach because many other reasons for insomnia exist, such as inflammation (pain), food allergies, anxiety, toxicity (chemical overload) and emotional stress. Finding the blockages or deficiencies in the serotonin pathway, and all other pathways, is always the best approach.

HAPPY OR HORMONAL? – CIRCULATION/SEX 1

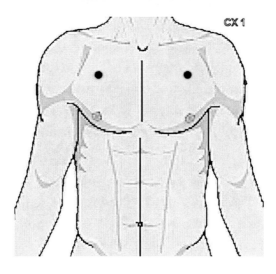

Figure 14: Circulation Sex 1

Related Neurotransmitter: Glutamate or Aspartate (high levels)

Organ or System: Reproductive System & Hormones

Main Biomarkers: Cholesterol, Progesterone, Testosterone, Estrogens

Common Hormetic Nutrients: Iron, Niacin (B3), Sulfur, Pantothenic Acid (B5), Zinc, Pfaffia Paniculata (suma herb)

No woman, or teenage boy, on earth needs a doctor to tell them hormones are powerful. These specialized proteins are responsible for a large percentage of the chemical reactions taking place in the body at any given moment. When the hormones related to reproduction drift or are forced out of balance, the PEP circulation/sex 1 (CX 1) becomes detectable with FBA. CX 1 is located roughly half way between the nipple and the collarbone.

Hormonal imbalances are the result of many factors, including glandular dysfunction, liver congestion, allergic reactions, fungal and other microbial infections, birth control pills, poor diet (blood sugar problems)

and toxicity from environmental causes, such as pesticides and plastics. FBA and lifestyle adjustments can successfully treat all these situations, addressed in detail throughout *Hope for Health*.

Hormones exemplify the interconnectedness of the body as a whole. If any become unbalanced, a myriad of symptoms may develop including the following ones:

- Blood sugar problems
- Breast tenderness
- Depression
- Edema
- Endometriosis
- Fibrocystic breasts
- Hot flashes
- Infertility
- Irregular menstrual cycles
- Loss of libido
- Osteoporosis
- PMS
- Poly Cystic Ovarian Syndrome
- Unexplained weight gain[276]
- Uterine fibroids

Looking at the figure below and observing all the arrows pointing in different directions, gives an indication of the complexity of the hormonal system. Any one of these arrows represents a place where a breakdown can occur. The body relies on hormetic nutrients at these same locations to keep the hormones flowing correctly.

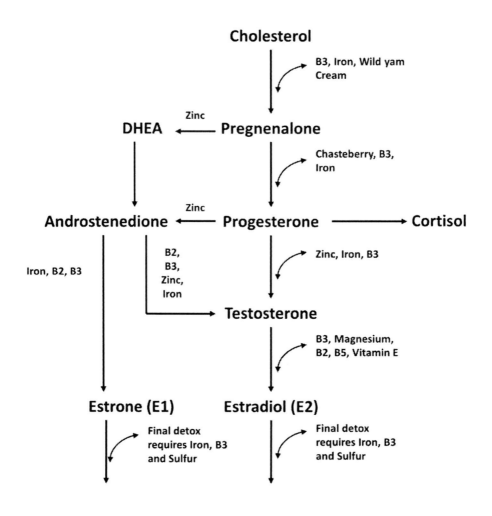

Figure 15: Hormone Pathway

HORMONE REPLACEMENT THERAPY (HRT)

Hormones are extremely complicated substances with powerful effects on the tissues they target. So powerful, in fact, out-of-whack hormones are both the cause of, and the result of, many functional problems. Knowing this, many books have been written espousing the benefits of hormone replacement therapy (HRT) to keep the body young, strong, and wrinkle-free. The practice of giving replacement hormones when they are low in the body is, on the surface, logically sound. However, digging a little deeper reveals a few potential problems.

First, this approach does nothing to correct the reasons why the hormones were low (or high) in the first place. Second, since the process of hormonal production and release is dependent upon numerous feedback loops, adding hormones into this delicate system is almost guaranteed to be problematic, leading to states of hormone resistance or pituitary suppression. HRT in these cases would only make the situation worse. It is far wiser to do everything possible to reestablish the normal ebb and flow of hormone production, release, and breakdown before ever attempting HRT. FBA can do this.

In July of 2002, the National Institutes of Health (NIH) halted a large, in-progress study examining the effects of a widely used type of HRT medication called Prempro,® which combines the hormones estrogen and progestin. The NIH took action because the hormones increased a woman's risk of breast cancer, as well as heart disease, blood clots, and stroke. The findings were published in *JAMA*, the Journal of the American Medical Association. A review of preliminary data found a 26 percent increase in breast cancer, a 29 percent increase in heart attacks, and a 22 percent increase in total cardiovascular disease among women receiving the hormones compared with women who received a placebo. Three months later, a British HRT study was also stopped for essentially the same reasons. There had been hopes HRT could reduce the risk of coronary heart disease, but the reverse appears to be true.

These results are not at all surprising to many operating in the realm of natural medicine. In fact, doctors have known for almost 30 years that estrogen replacement by itself increased the likelihood of some cancers. That's why both of the aborted studies above combined artificial progesterone along with estrogen. Even this combination together was not enough to prevent significant side effects. Proponents of HRT use compounds consisting of non-synthetic, bio-identical hormones similar to the ones made within the body. This is a valid point. When the body requires hormones, it needs natural hormones, not the synthetic version. However, there is more to the story.

Natural hormone replacement can be very useful in some instances, such as after a hysterectomy, thyroidectomy, or other surgeries that require the removal of hormone-producing tissue; when an autoimmune or congenital disease has damaged hormonal tissues; or when exhausted hormone-regulating glands need a short-term break. In these cases, a doctor must regularly monitor the replacement hormones to prevent the unwanted effect of too much hormone, called hormone resistance.

BIRTH CONTROL PILLS

Hormone replacements in the form of birth control pills are one of the worst abuses of medicine in recent history. When considering birth control pills, a basic understanding of the intricate arrangement of hormones; their impressive power over metabolism, mood, and memory; and their response to negative influences of diet and stress, should produce more than a pause or a mere red flag. For a medical doctor to prescribe birth control pills to a young girl with menstrual cramps and presume that he has acted in her best interest shows his absolute ignorance of the sensitivity within the endocrine system. He has, in fact, set her on a course that is potentially life altering in the most negative sense. From a natural perspective, the belief that artificially controlling the most basic and fundamental cycle of womanhood and expecting mild or no consequences is in utter contrast to the fundamentals of logic and reason. One need only ask friends and neighbors if they know any young women with ovarian cysts, fibroid tumors, endometriosis, or who are having difficulty getting pregnant. If they know any pre-menopausal women taking anti-depressants, thyroid medication, or sleep aids, there is a good chance these women took the birth control pill at some point in their lives. All these issues are hormonally related and connected to the female menstrual cycle.

Birth control pills are generally one of two types. The first type keeps estrogen high so the follicle-stimulating hormone and luteinizing hormone peaks don't happen (explained below). This prevents an egg from developing properly or prevents ovulation all together. The second type keeps progesterone high so the body thinks it's pregnant, thereby not releasing additional eggs.

The Effects of Birth Control Pills

- They confuse the body's natural hormonal production, which in the very least will eventually make menopause difficult.

- They can create fibroid tumors. Many times fibroid tumors spontaneously go away at menopause because of a drop in estrogen.

- They lower vitamin B6 levels, which can lead to depression, food allergies, carpal tunnel syndrome, and sensitivities to electromagnetic fields.

- They can affect fertility.

- They can result in recurrent yeast infections.

- They can lead to other known problems, including excessive uterine bleeding, blood clots, hypertension, depression, vomiting, increased weight, kidney disease, and ovarian atrophy.

When told about the negative effects of birth control, women are often shocked and reply, "My doctor never told me that!" If a woman feels the need to use birth control pills at this time in her life, then, at a minimum, she should work with an FBA practitioner capable of monitoring the effects of the pills. Supporting her therapeutically in every way to help minimize the potential detrimental consequences of artificial hormone ingestion is a must.

THE FEMALE SEXUAL CYCLE

A key to understanding many of the issues women experience is to understand the female sexual cycle (menstrual cycle). Although there is variation with the normal length of the cycle, there should be certain trends before, during, and after ovulation. For instance, if a woman experiences unpleasant symptoms, such as uterine cramping, headaches, or bloating prior to ovulation, it is likely an issue with the hormone progesterone, which surges at these times. However, if a woman experiences the symptoms just prior to menstrual bleeding, estrogen imbalances are a stronger consideration.

The menstrual cycle should be a rhythmic cycle lasting between 20 and 45 days, with an optimal cycle lasting 28 days. Its purpose is to prepare a female's egg (ovum) for fertilization with a male's sperm and to prepare the uterus to receive and sustain the fertilized egg.

There are three different hierarchies of hormones to consider when discussing the female sexual cycle. The first comes from the hypothalamus and is the gonadotropin-releasing hormone (GnRH). Its job is to stimulate the anterior portion of the pituitary gland—the gland in charge of overseeing the entire cycle. The anterior pituitary gland releases two important hormones: follicle stimulating hormone (FSH) and luteinizing hormone (LH). These two then act directly on the ovaries, encouraging them to secrete estrogen and progesterone, respectively.

Most consider day one to be the first day of menstrual bleeding. This day is actually the end of some very important steps, as seen in the following graph.

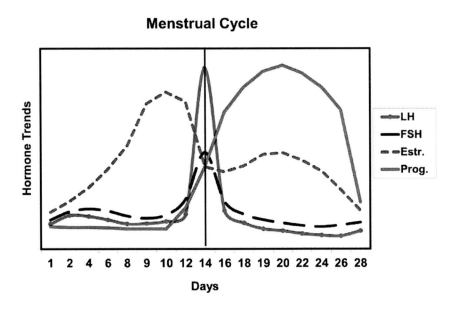

Figure 16: Female Menstrual Cycle

Synopsis

- Day 1: Shedding of uterine lining with increases in estrogen from days 1 through 12.

- Day 12: Marked increase in FSH, drastic increase in LH, estrogen at its peak.

- Day 13: Dramatic drop in estrogen initiates ovulation.

- Day 14: Ovulation, FSH and LH at their peak, progesterone rising.

- Day 13: Surge in progesterone until day 23.

- Day 15: Drop in FSH and LH.

- Day 23: Progesterone at its peak.

- Day 24: Drop in progesterone until day 28.

- Day 28: lowest levels of progesterone initiates the shedding of the uterine lining (menstrual bleeding) and the cycle repeats.

Ovulation

Ovulation is the moment when one ovary releases an egg. At birth, a woman has around one million eggs in both ovaries. Each month, after the onset of puberty, an egg contest begins. The body allows 6 to 12 eggs to participate in the contest, but only one is the winner. Under the influence of follicle stimulating hormone (FSH), a follicle will contain each contestant. One follicle will become dominant and cause the others to die off (become atretic). Thus the winner, the sole remaining follicle, will mature and eventually burst at the time of ovulation, releasing the egg within, now called an ovum.

For a woman with a 28-day cycle, ovulation occurs 14 days after the onset of menstruation. The first part of a woman's sexual cycle may vary from month to month by a few days; however, the last half of the cycle, from the time of ovulation to just before the start of menses, is usually a consistent 14 days. There are five characteristics of ovulation:

1. The rapid growth of the follicle by FSH.
2. Decreasing amounts of estrogen.
3. Increasing amounts of progesterone to promote pregnancy.
4. Release of the egg from the follicle.
5. A surge of LH to produce a corpus luteum.

Corpus Luteum

After ovulation, the winning egg receives her crown. A cloud of granulosa cells, called a *corona radiata*, surround the ovum. LH, which aids in implantation, surges 6 to 10 fold two days before ovulation, transforming the granulosa cells into lutein cells. The corpus luteum is the combination of the ovum and the lutein cells. Over the next 6 to 12 days, the corpus luteum will grow, secreting progesterone and some estrogen while awaiting fertilization. If none occurs, the estrogen secretions soon shut off both LH and FSH, and the corpus luteum involutes or dies.

Estrogen

This is perhaps the most talked about hormone in the female cycle. It is responsible for the sexual characteristics of the female and causes the proliferation of many reproductive cells. Its job during the sexual cycle is to prepare the ovum for fertilization. Estrogen is high during the early part of the cycle and drops at ovulation. Too much estrogen is sometimes a cause for failed conception or can result in a failure to ovulate.

One of the most common gynecological problems is irregular menstrual cycles. Skipping periods, heavy bleeding, and spotting are all menstrual irregularities. When estrogen levels are high, the lining of the uterus builds up in an exaggerated manner. This overproduction leads to a dramatic release of tissue at the time of menstruation, and heavy bleeding results. Too much estrogen is usually associated with cramping, a shorter cycle, and a longer period. Higher progesterone levels, on the other hand, usually mean light bleeding with little pain and a longer cycle.

When the overall levels of estrogen are low, the uterine lining never properly forms, and frequent release, or spotting, is likely. Too little estrogen results in vaginal dryness in some women and hot flashes in women during menopause.

Progesterone "Pro Gestation"

Progesterone is the hormone most responsible for the healthy development of a baby. Many women who have trouble maintaining a pregnancy usually need to increase progesterone. Its functions during the sexual cycle include raising body temperature (incubation), preparing the uterus for pregnancy and the breasts for lactation, and inhibiting FSH and LH. If fertilization does not occur, progesterone drops, initiating menstrual bleeding due to the shedding of the uterine lining. If fertilization does occur, then a hormone called human chorionic gonadotropin (HCG) prevents progesterone from decreasing. HCG is the hormone detected on a pregnancy test. With fertilization, HCG will be present in the urine and blood stream around one week after ovulation.

Pre Menstrual Syndrome

Researchers who study PMS estimate that as many as 40 percent of women suffer from this condition at some point in their lives. Bloating, acne, pain, emotional changes (moodiness, anger, depression), and fatigue are some of the common symptoms of PMS. Technically, in order to have PMS, the symptoms must occur at the same time each month. For example, if a patient's symptoms relate to high progesterone, the symptoms would occur near the middle of the cycle. Most PMS symptoms, however, relate to excess estrogen and would therefore occur prior to menstrual bleeding.

The Causes of Hormonal Imbalances

1. *Poor diet* – A poor diet, those high in refined and processed foods, disrupts digestion, which leads to inflammation of the linings of the small intestine. An irritated lining leads to poor absorption of nutrients (leaky gut syndrome). Poor absorption of nutrients leads to inadequate resources for the breakdown and processing of hormones and promotes the overgrowth of unwanted organisms, such as Candida.

2. *Plastic and pesticides* (xenoestrogens) – Plastics and pesticides that are absorbed into our bodies act like estrogens. In lakes with large amounts of pesticides, fish become hermaphroditic, newborn alligators are all female, and the male alligators become feminized.

3. *Meats and milk* – This is another source of exogenous hormonal compounds with estrogen-like qualities. Last year 750,000 cows received injections of bovine growth hormone and antibiotics. Ranches often use pesticide-laden, genetically modified feed for cattle.

4. *Liver congestion* – The liver is the organ that does all the breaking down of used hormones. If the liver is congested (full, fatigued, overworked), it does not have the resources to detoxify female hormones. As a result, the excess hormones continue to float

freely in the blood stream, interacting with estrogen receptors on various tissues and creating a hormonal overload. See the chapter *Arthritic or Toxic?* for more details.

5. *Fungal infections* – There is a strong relationship between fungal infections and estrogen imbalances. Fungus, like Candida Albicans, thrive in estrogen-dominant women, altering the normally smooth increases and decreases of estrogen throughout the cycle. See the chapter *Infection or Autoimmunity?* for more details.

6. *Adrenal fatigue* – The adrenal glands are a secondary producer of estrogen. Messages from the pituitary gland force the adrenals to make more. However, tired adrenals cannot meet the demand, so the ovaries work overtime. Again, this means more peaks and valleys for estrogen.

7. *Allergies* – Allergens generate numerous amounts of immune system chemicals, increase inflammation in the tissues, and increase water retention and bloating, all of which make detoxification of the reproductive hormones by the liver more difficult. See the chapter *Allergies or Inflammation?* for details.

8. *Medications* – Birth control pills and hormone replacement therapy (HRT), designed to correct imbalances, often create many of their own.

9. *Nutritional Imbalances* – Proper quality and quantity of nutrients must be present in order for detoxification to take place effectively. Every illness has a deficiency in hormetic nutrients. Without proper nutrition, hormonal imbalances won't be the only thing wrong.

10. *Stress* – This is a powerful disrupter of hormonal balance and leads to a myriad of unwanted effects, such as weight gain, sleep disruptions, adrenal gland fatigue, osteoporosis, and more. See the chapter *Tired or Stressed?* for details.

ANDROPAUSE – MALE MENOPAUSE

Traditionally, doctors did not consider age-related male hormone changes to be problematic because fertility in men persists until an advanced age. By contrast, ovarian failure in women results in significant hormonal drops well before these same hormonal decreases occur in men. However, the male still experiences plenty of the signs progressive age-related hormonal change, including:

- Decrease in libido
- Decrease in erectile function
- Spells of mental fatigue
- Inability to concentrate
- Episodes of depression
- Muscle soreness
- Decrease in physical stamina
- Unexplained weight gain
- Increase in fat distribution around chest and hips
- Sweating attacks
- Emotional episodes

The changes above usually begin in the fourth and fifth decades as androgens diminish. Androgens are hormones like testosterone that predominantly encourage masculine characteristics. Many consider androgen deficiencies as the male equivalent of menopause, called Andropause.

Testosterone production in males is predominantly the responsibility of the testicles. The same pituitary sex hormones that are responsible for female characteristics and ovum development in women also stimulate and regulate testosterone release and sperm production in men. Specifically, luteinizing hormone (LH) stimulates testosterone production in the testicles. This process is under negative feedback, meaning the higher the testosterone levels, the lower the LH secretions and vice versa. Follicle stimulating hormone (FSH) and testosterone encourage the production of sperm.

As discussed above, hormone replacement for women is a last-resort option; and when used indiscriminately, makes a bad situation even worse. The same is true for men. Excessive use of androgens (testosterone, androstenedione, DHEA, and testosterone derivatives) can activate subclinical prostatic tumors that are androgen-dependent. By the age of 70, at least 50 percent of men have subclinical prostate cancer, which is especially susceptible to growth stimulation by androgens.

Men will encounter problems when estrogen levels increase as well. The most likely culprit for increased estrogen and decreased testosterone in men is a blood sugar imbalance, specifically, insulin resistance.[277] Testosterone in these men is converted to estrogen via an enzyme called aromatase.[278] Unaware of this, men with low testosterone will seek help from their primary care physician. Not a good idea. In all likelihood, the traditional doctor will do a blood test to measure testosterone levels and discover that the hormone is low. So far, so good. Next he will prescribe a testosterone cream to boost the low levels.[279] The cream, he is told, is to be rubbed into the fatty areas such as the belly and buttocks. Uh-oh, here comes trouble. The fatty areas are where aromatase is found in the greatest concentration. Soon after applying the testosterone, it immediately undergoes a transformation by aromatase into estrogen. The long term negative effects of this course of action are predictable.

The conversion of testosterone into estrogen via aromatase is not 100%. This means that at the start of treatment the patient may in fact feel better as some testosterone gets into the blood stream. The honeymoon, however, does not last long. Usually within eight weeks or less, estrogen is present in abundance, leaving the patient worse off than when he started. Now, not only are his symptoms the same or worse, but he has a whole new issue to contend with – the detoxification of estrogen. Not to mention that insulin resistance, the metabolic state responsible for creating low testosterone levels in the first place, has not yet been addressed.

Testing For Hormones

FBA allows the practitioner to determine whether hormones are high, low, or just right. It cannot however, tell exactly what those levels are. Thankfully, blood, saliva, and urine tests can help evaluate hormones in both women and men. Measurements of hormonal levels are important, since they provide a baseline—the mark from which a practitioner can determine therapeutic progress.

Saliva testing reflects the active tissue concentrations (free fractions), while blood analysis contains a total of both the active and inactive (protein bound) hormones. Urine contains active hormones, as well as the broken down substances of detoxified hormones called metabolites. Each of these different tests has its own diagnostic value. Since saliva testing reveals how much hormone is actually working (active) as opposed to just the total amount present, saliva is generally the superior assessment for hormones.

Practitioners can test the following six primary hormones through the basic male salivary profile:

1. *DHEA* – This is the precursor for both male and female hormones. It is an anti- stress hormone produced by the adrenal glands. Unmonitored intake can easily alter the delicate balance between hormones.

2. *Androstenedione* – This is a weak male hormone (androgen) and a precursor of both male and female hormones. Unmonitored intake in men can cause excessive female hormone production with minimal male hormone production. In women, unmonitored intake usually causes excess male hormone production with body and facial hair stimulation.

3. *Testosterone* – This is the main testicular androgen and is a precursor to the highly potent dihydrotestosterone male hormone. Excessive amounts of testosterone promote hardening of the blood vessels, aggression, and prostate problems. They also increase total cholesterol.

4. *Dihydrotestosterone (DHT)* – This hormone is made from testosterone in certain tissues. The level of free active progesterone controls the rate of DHT production. Excess DHT causes prostate enlargement and thinning of scalp hair.

5. *Progesterone* – This hormone is important in both sexes. It is a natural calming agent to the nervous system. It also keeps in check excessive DHT production (a downstream hormone from testosterone) and counterbalances the effects of excessive estrone. Unmonitored intake can lead to breast enlargement, depression, and weight gain.[280] In many women, it can help prevent cancer.[281] [282]

6. Estrone – This is an estrogen that both sexes produce in the fat cells. The more fat, the more estrone, which itself in turn promotes fat deposits. The hormone androstenedione produces estrone. Excess of estrone can cause breast enlargement and may contribute to prostate enlargement. In males, a certain low level of estrone is mandatory to balance the androgens.

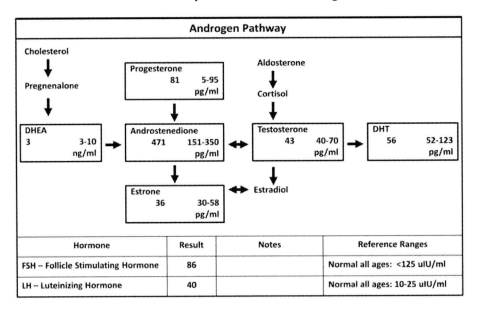

Figure 17: Saliva Test for Male Hormones

Blockages resulting in the symptoms of Andropause can occur anywhere within the hormonal stream. From the test results on the previous page, one can see that testosterone is on the low end of normal while its precursor androstenedione is too high. This is a prime example of beavers in the river. A dam between these two important male hormones is blocking the one downstream, making testosterone deficient. The hormetic nutrients B2, B3, zinc, and iron are important for correcting this problem.

FBA for Andropause

Knowing a person's color type (Red, Green or Blue) is important for balancing hormones. For Blue men, copper tends to be a commonly needed mineral. It is not one of the primary nutrients required to detoxify and utilize hormones, but it does work in cooperation with those that are, such as iron and zinc. Green men will need extra magnesium and Reds will require vitamin B12, B6 or folic acid. Several other hormetic nutrients will undoubtedly be necessary in order to fully balance the altered hormonal state and to stabilize any other dysregulated systems. These will be found one by one in their order of importance with FBA.

FUELED OR FATTY? – GALL BLADDER 1

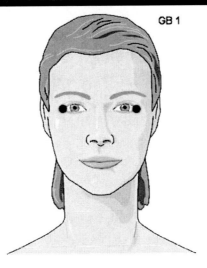

Figure 18: Gall Bladder 1

Related Neurotransmitter: Acetylcholine (low levels)

Organ or System: Gall Bladder

Main Biomarkers: Cholesterol, HDL, LDL, Homocysteine, C-Reactive Protein

Common Hormetic Nutrients: Niacin (B3), Taurine, Pantothenic Acid (B5), Fat Soluble Vitamins, Essential Fatty Acids

The gall bladder is a specialized organ adjacent to the liver. Its job is to store a fat-busting substance called bile. The gall bladder squeezes bile into the small intestine whenever a meal containing fat enters this part of the digestive tract. Like dish soap in a greasy pan, bile breaks down, or emulsifies, fats on contact. Irritation of the gall bladder is a common problem, occurring with the ingestion of too much fat or too many inflammatory fats, such as trans fats and heated vegetable oils. Combining these unhealthy oils with sugars and processed flour (just think dessert), is nearly a guarantee of future digestive trouble. Gall bladder stress activates the PEP GB 1, located at the outermost corner of the eyes.

Although fats have a bad reputation, people should not excommunicate them from the diet. Fats are essential for energy; cell membranes; producing *all* hormones and other hormone-like substances; activating fat-soluble vitamins, such as vitamins A, D, and E; and for high brain performance. Despite all of its benefits, people often consider fat to be unhealthy because of its association with cholesterol, the espoused cause of heart disease. But there is much more to the story.

CHOLESTEROL & TRIGLYCERIDES

In traditional medicine, doctors base heart attack prevention on an ever-changing effort to place subjects into low, moderate, and high risk categories all based upon different types and fractions of the cholesterol molecule. Researchers have established scales and guidelines to promote this effort. However, there is very little evidence to support the contention that a diet low in cholesterol and saturated fat actually reduces death from heart disease or in any way increases one's life span. Before a discussion of the true causes of heart disease can begin, a detailed look at the campaign against high cholesterol is necessary.

Cholesterol is a steroid normally present in every cell of the body and is essential to life. Cholesterol is part of the membrane of all cells, works to build and repair cells, and produces hormones, such as estrogen and testosterone. Its main job, however, is for the liver to convert it into cholic acid (up to 80 percent of all cholesterol becomes cholic acid). Cholic acid combines with other substances in the liver to produce bile salts, which the gall bladder stores to aid in the digestion and absorption of fat. The body produces about 70 to 80 percent of its own cholesterol. Only 20 to 30 percent of cholesterol comes from the diet.[283]

The American Heart Association recommends that all persons 20 years of age or older have a lipid profile performed every five years.[284] The lipid profile is the measurement of the different types of cholesterol and the triglyceride levels. Most traditionally trained doctors would agree to the following things:

- Total cholesterol below 200 mg/dl is good, and anything over 240 mg/dl is bad.

- LDL cholesterol should measure below 130 mg/dl.

- HDL cholesterol should range between 35 and 40 mg/dl.

- If the HDL cholesterol reaches 60 mg/dl or higher, a person has a reduced chance for a heart attack.

- Triglycerides should be less than 200 mg/dl.

Many complementary doctors who work in the functional realm evaluate these numbers in the following way:

- Total cholesterol should range from 150 to 220 mg/dl.

- HDL (the "good" cholesterol) should be at least 25 percent of the total cholesterol.

- LDL should be less than 120 mg/dl.

- Triglycerides should be less than 50 percent of the total cholesterol.

The triglyceride level, not cholesterol, is often a better predictor of heart disease than other markers. Triglycerides are a particular form of fat that the blood transports to a needed tissue. Triglycerides make up the majority of the body fat. Triglycerides in the blood, or serum, come from food or from the liver. After consuming a meal containing fat, the intestines will package some of the excess and transport it via blood vessels to the liver. Once the liver receives the fats, it then takes fatty acids released by adipose tissue, or fat cells, and bundles them up as triglycerides, which the rest of the body may use as fuel. Here are two patient examples:

Patient A:	Total cholesterol:	280 (above normal)
	LDL:	175
	HDL:	70
	Triglycerides:	130

Patient B:	Total cholesterol:	180 (normal)
	LDL:	97
	HDL:	35
	Triglycerides:	165

Traditional doctors would strongly consider Patient A for pharmaceutical intervention, but is this person really in trouble? It is true that the total cholesterol is above the normal range; however, the HDL number is greater than 25 percent, and the triglycerides are less than 50 percent. This patient actually has a good balance of all the lipid levels.

Patient B, on the other hand, is within normal limits on all the levels. However, the triglycerides are more than 50 percent of the total cholesterol, and the HDL is less than 25 percent of total cholesterol. Patient B is actually at greater risk for a heart attack even though the measurements are within the standard normal limits.

Why Cholesterol is High?

At least four understood reasons can cause an elevated cholesterol level:

1. The body is producing too much cholesterol;

2. A person is eating too much cholesterol in the diet;

3. The body is not breaking down cholesterol properly, resulting in nutritional deficiency; or

4. One or more hormone-producing tissues, usually the thyroid or pituitary is under (hypo) functioning.

The most common of these four is that the body is not properly breaking down cholesterol.

In the previous chapter, the chart of hormonal production included cholesterol. If cholesterol is the precursor to all other hormones, what would happen to the hormones if cholesterol was lowered? All of the body's important reproductive hormones would decrease as well! This is precisely what happens when patients take cholesterol-lowering drugs, like statins.

THE TRUE CAUSE OF HEART DISEASE - INFLAMMATION

Doctors who cling to the shibboleth, "High cholesterol is the cause of heart disease," continue to look for more sophisticated ways to measure the cholesterol molecule. The NMR LipoProfile,[285] for example, uses the principle of natural resonance, breaks cholesterol down into 15 specific kinds of lipoprotein subclasses.[286] [287] Likewise, the Vertical Auto Profile or VAP Test also measures 15 fractions, but it does so through high-speed centrifugation, separating cholesterol apart into smaller and smaller bits.[288] Many assume that the more doctors understand about cholesterol, the more the links between it and heart disease will be. But there are major problems with the cholesterol-heart disease connection.

Approximately half of all patients who develop clogged arteries, called coronary heart disease (CHD), have normal or only marginal elevations in total and LDL (bad) cholesterol levels.[289] [290] Conversely, a significant number of people with elevated cholesterol never develop CHD. These facts illuminate an approach that is missing the mark. Instead of looking beyond cholesterol for the cause of CHD, pharmaceutical medicine chose to tighten its guidelines, lowering "bad" cholesterol (LDL) from 130 to less than 100. This, of course, led to greater sales of cholesterol-lowering drugs, called statins. Statin drugs, which prevent an enzyme necessary for cholesterol formation from working, riddle the person with nasty side effects, including liver toxicity and severe muscle pain.[291] These medicines do in fact lower cholesterol; but one must ask the following question: Do they help prevent heart attacks? In 20 to 40 percent of people taking statins, the answer is no.[292] [293] [294]

The main question for heart attack prevention is, "How do we stop arteries from clogging?" Clogged arteries are the result of the buildup of atherosclerotic plaques. These are not just cholesterol-based deposits. They are comprised of numerous components, including smooth muscle cells, calcium, connective tissue, white blood cells, cholesterol, and fatty acids. The growth of plaques begins *inside* the artery wall, between the inner and outer layers. But why? With a scrape or a cut on the skin, the body protects the injured area by forming a hard scab. This wall of defense prevents further damage while the body heals the torn tissue. Likewise, plaques acts as internal scabs, laid down by the body to protect damaged or weakened arteries. Why are they damaged? If researchers could answer this question, they would know the cause of heart disease. Alternative practitioners know the cause and the answer: Excess inflammation damages the arteries.

C-reactive protein (CRP) is a substance that serves as a marker for inflammation inside the body, especially the arteries. CRP has attracted a great deal of attention ever since a large study published in the New England Journal of Medicine in 2002 suggested that this protein was a significantly better predictor of future cardiovascular events than LDL cholesterol.[295] A second study published three years later, examined the relationship between statin use, CRP levels, and subsequent coronary event rates. Regardless of the levels of LDL cholesterol, patients who had low CRP levels had better clinical outcomes.[296] In other words, those who were less inflamed had fewer heart attacks.[297]

Measuring the blood levels for cholesterol - the lipid profile - is still a good idea because any additional data about one's health is never bad. However, to assess the risk of heart disease, it is critical to include blood levels of the inflammatory chemical C-reactive protein, along with two others, homocysteine and fibrinogen. Homocysteine is strongly correlated with heart disease and is discussed at length in the chapter *Panic or Pass Out?*

Several factors, including infections, trauma, and toxicity, can cause inflammation. In life, these are usually temporary states. The chronically inflamed person, however, most likely got that way because of his or her diet. Heated oils, processed grains, and refined sugars are the troublesome food trio most responsible for systemic inflammation.

The American Heart Association recommends a low saturated fat diet and the liberal use of vegetable oils.[298] But there is a problem. Many cultures, including Eskimos and the Masai tribes of Africa, eat saturated fat as their primary food but have low or no heart disease.[299] So what does this mean?

All fats are not created equal. Man-made synthetic and processed fats (trans fats) interfere with cholesterol breakdown, and should be avoided. The process of partial hydrogenation changes the shapes of natural fats and oils so they interfere with, rather than promote, normal fat metabolism. According to a study published in the New England Journal of Medicine, it has been estimated that by simply eliminating trans fats from the U.S. food supply could prevent between 6 and 19 percent of heart attacks and related deaths, or more than 200,000 each year.[300]

These processed fats are in nearly everything people buy in the grocery store, from salad dressings to candy bars, and from chips to breads. Partially hydrogenated fats and oils block the normal conversion of cholesterol in the liver, causing an elevation of cholesterol in the blood. Margarine, which is often touted for its lack of cholesterol, is produced from partially hydrogenated fats. One of the biggest cases of misinformation in recent history is the suggestion that eating margarine instead of butter will reduce cholesterol. It is true that butter contains cholesterol and that margarine does not. But, butter also contains high levels of normal fat mobilizing nutrients. It is a whole food designed to take care of its own fats if eaten in moderation. Margarine can actually increase cholesterol levels and heart attacks.[301]

The same facts are true for eggs. Egg yolks are one of the highest sources of cholesterol. But they are also one of the highest sources of natural fat mobilizers. Eggs and butter are two examples of whole foods, which research shows are actually useful for lowering cholesterol and improving fat metabolism.[302] [303] Only patients who have severely elevated cholesterol, such as those who have a family history of poor fat metabolism and breakdown, should avoid them.

So why would the American Heart Association recommend a low saturated fat diet? Misguided ideas have led to people barring saturated fats like butter from the dinner table. But most of the fat found in clogged arteries is not saturated, it is polyunsaturated. Polyunsaturated oils are the inflammatory ones and include corn, soy, safflower, and canola oils—the very same oils recommended by the American Heart Association. These fats tend to become oxidized or rancid when exposed to heat through cooking. [304] [305] Oxidation is one of the most aggressive forms of tissue inflammation and is the reason why antioxidants, such as those found in fresh vegetables are the cornerstone of an anti-inflammatory diet and therefore an important part of heart disease prevention.[306]

Remember, the primary goal when trying to prevent heart attacks is inflammation reduction. Saturated fat by itself is neutral or can be anti-inflammatory, but not when combined with sugars.[307] [308] Americans love sweets and grease. In the Standard American Diet, rarely will saturated fat be unaccompanied by copious amounts of sugar. With each dessert, Americans increase their risk for heart disease,[309] [310] eating roughly 150 pounds of refined sweeteners each year.[311]

The rise in CHD to America's #1 killer began around 1920 and continues to the present. During the same period, the percentage of dietary vegetable oils in the form of margarine, shortening, and refined oils increased nearly 400 percent while the consumption of sugar and processed foods increased about 60 percent.[312] Studies from around the world have consistently demonstrated that in populations where the diet was high in sugar, processed flours, and heated vegetable oils, deaths from all manner of disease, including heart disease, are much higher.[313] [314] [315] [316] [317]

FBA FOR HEART DISEASE

FBA can do a great deal to help lower the risk of heart disease. By using the inflammatory biomarkers C-reactive protein, homocysteine, and fibrinogen, an FBA practitioner can discover the type of inflammatory process and the hormetic nutrients needed to stop it.

Perhaps the primary goal of heart disease prevention is to avoid any lifestyle or dietary pattern that promotes blood sugar instability. Managing glucose effectively results in an abundance of energy and low levels of inflammation. As described in the chapter, *Hypoglycemia or Histamine* and in Appendix C, *Energy to Burn*, the body has three choices when wanting to reduce extra blood sugar (glucose).

1. Convert it to fat;

2. Store it as glycogen; or

3. Make more triglycerides (a sugar molecule attached to three fatty acids).

These three options directly relate to the dysfunctions defining metabolic syndrome: high blood pressure, insulin resistance (high insulin and high blood sugar), elevated triglycerides, and being overweight.

Glucose is also critical for the formation of all soft tissues, such as ligaments and cartilage. Excess glucose, along with the inflammation it generates, has a direct negative impact on the joints, which is one reason why so many people in their middle years begin to complain of joint pain.

Nutritional factors that help to balance glucose, lower cholesterol, reduce inflammation, and consequently lower the risk for heart disease include adequate levels of vitamins A and C; specific B vitamins, especially niacinamide (B3); magnesium, zinc, and chromium; trace elements, which can increase the levels of HDL; and fat mobilizing substances, including choline, taurine and betaine.

Although patterns do emerge, each person's hormetic nutrient profile will be unique. The beauty of FBA is that it can find which specific nutrients a person may need. Beyond the hormetic nutrients, lifestyle considerations are essential. Good digestive health; a proper diet full of anti-inflammatory fats, antioxidant-rich foods, and unheated oils; along with proper exercise are critical, not only for reducing the risk for heart disease but for improved health in general. These topics are discussed throughout *Hope for Health.*

PANIC OR PASS OUT? – HEART 1

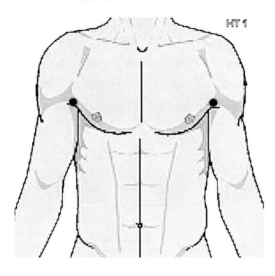

Figure 19: Heart 1

Related Neurotransmitter: Norepinephrine (high levels)

Organ or System: Heart

Main Biomarkers: Homocysteine, C-reactive Protein

Common Hormetic Nutrients: Thiamin (B1), Riboflavin (B2), Potassium, Magnesium

The heart is the most active muscle in the body, beating an average of 100,000 times per day and circulating nearly 4,300 gallons of blood in that time.[318] Since the heart is a muscle, it will have the same mineral requirements as any other muscle. Contraction is dependent upon calcium, while muscle relaxation requires magnesium.[319] Potassium is also very important, since it, along with sodium, aids in the transport of all materials into and out of the cells through a mechanism called the sodium-potassium pump.[320]

When it comes to functional problems, the body, as expected, will send some sort of distress signal. For muscles, cramps or spasms are common.

Cramps or spasms in the foot, lower leg, spinal muscles or eyelids, usually reveal that the body is deficient in one of the important muscle-minerals mentioned above. This warning should not be ignored. If muscles are indicating they have unmet needs, it is likely that the heart does as well. Palpitations, or flutters of the heart, are a sure confirmation, signifying a person needs immediate help.

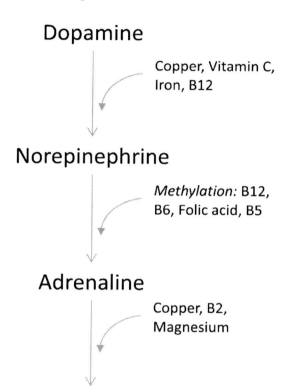

Dopamine

Copper, Vitamin C, Iron, B12

Norepinephrine

Methylation: B12, B6, Folic acid, B5

Adrenaline

Copper, B2, Magnesium

The neurotransmitter associated with the PEP Heart 1 is norepinephrine, an excitatory chemical generated by the stress response. When stress has persisted for too long, or the body no longer has the resources to break down the chemicals of stress, Heart 1, located just inside the armpit, becomes activated. A prolonged fight-or-flight response is a dangerous physical state. Spikes of norepinephrine can cause heart attacks and heart attack-like symptoms even by taking over-the-counter cold remedies that contain norepinephrine in a synthetic form.[321] Supplying the necessary hormetic nutrients required to break norepinerphrine down can reduce its levels in the body. However, since norepinephrine is the result of an ongoing stress response, managing this undesirable state becomes a principal goal. The chapters *Tired or Stressed?* and *The Fountain of Youth & Anti-Aging?*, provide the knowledge and practical steps necessary to manage and reduce the deadly stress response.

BLOOD PRESSURE

High blood pressure, or hypertension, is the most common primary diagnosis in America, leading to 35 million office visits.[322] Hypertension affects one third of all people over 20 years of age [323] and results in roughly 40 million Americans taking daily anti-hypertensive medication.[324] To achieve the goal of blood pressure less than 140/90, most patients will require two or more prescriptions.[325] To top it off, lifelong dependency on blood pressure medications is the norm and results in repeat doctor visits, ongoing medical expenses and a heftier bottom line for the pharmaceutical industry. Worst of all, dependence on medication may leave patients trapped and unempowered by medicine's single-minded approach.

High blood pressure may be the clearest example of a functional problem made worse by traditional pharmaceutical management. Why? Because it fails to address its causes such as:

- Dehydration
- Inflammation
- Insulin resistance
- Toxicity
- Nervousness
- Autonomic nervous system imbalance
- Food allergies
- Nutritional imbalances
- Kidney stress

- Arteriosclerosis

The causes listed above are, for the most part, temporary and correctable. Those that aren't, such as arteriosclerosis, have taken a long time to develop, while others may be congenital in nature, but these represent a small minority. Therefore, for the vast majority of hypertension cases, FBA practitioners can use straightforward, non-invasive, functional approaches to reduce or normalize high blood pressure. Realizing this, another thought comes to mind: Since high blood pressure is a sign that something is wrong, not a disease in itself, is high blood pressure always bad? In the short term, could it actually be necessary?

If the body is toxic, it naturally increases blood pressure in order to filter toxins more quickly through the kidneys and the liver. If the body is dehydrated, blood pressure increases so thickened blood will travel through the vessels faster, ensuring the same amount of oxygen and nutrients reach target tissues in a timely manner. Food allergies and inflammation both raise blood pressure levels, as well. Therefore, raising blood pressure appears to be a necessary physiologic response in order to deal with a temporary imbalance or dysfunction.

This brings people to the billion dollar questions. If it is necessary for the body to alter blood pressure in order to combat a temporary ailment, wouldn't it be detrimental to lower it artificially with medications? Instead, wouldn't finding and fixing the cause of high blood pressure be the more prudent and health-promoting thing to do? Lastly, wouldn't it be best to do so sooner rather than later, before someone becomes twisted in a multi-drug chemical knot making the problem much harder to unwind?

Reasonable and rational scrutiny is unfortunately no match for a lifetime of medical programming. As if it were hypnotically implanted, when offered an alternative approach that would free them from their drug dependency, the expected response ensues, "But, I can't get off my blood pressure medicine." Perhaps they are right. First, a mission can't gain any ground if it starts with the words, "I can't." Second, lowering blood pressure often means changing one's current lifestyle, sometimes dramatically. People do not make dramatic changes unless absolutely compelled to do so, and even then it's fifty/fifty. Rare is the patient who is willing to do what is necessary to improve his health and not poison his body unnecessarily with medications; a salute to those reading this book.

Low Blood Pressure

Hypotension, or low blood pressure, is a rarely discussed condition, but one that is just as scary as any other heart-related problem. Feeling dizzy or lightheaded when getting up from a seated or lying down position are common complaints. Others include, temporary tunnel-like blindness, loss of peripheral vision, and passing out. Low blood pressure is not healthy. A sufficient amount of blood flow is necessary to supply the brain with oxygen and fuel. Those with low blood pressure tend to die earlier than those with normal or even high blood pressure.

Increasing blood pressure requires a coordinated effort between the heart, the adrenal glands and the thyroid. In order to not pass out when getting up from a resting supine position, blood vessels must rapidly constrict in response to chemical signals. Otherwise, the result is insufficient blood flow to the brain. Tired adrenal glands do not release adequate levels of a vessel-constricting hormone called adrenaline. Therefore, asking the question, "Do you feel lightheaded when standing up from a seated position?" is appropriate when evaluating adrenal gland health and function.

Sodium is the mineral deficiency most likely present with hypotension. Just as doctors recommend a low-salt diet for those with high blood pressure, extra salt is useful for those with low blood pressure. However, as with any mineral deficiency, it is important to evaluate its partner on the teeter-totter. In this case, potassium would be on the high side. For heart health, adrenal gland and thyroid support often becomes essential as well. Thankfully, following energetic pathways with FBA often leads straight to the problem, and the hormetic nutrients provide the solution.

Homocysteine

Another concern when Heart 1 is active is the presence of a highly inflammatory chemical called homocysteine. This chemical, discussed in the chapter *Fueled or Fatty?*, deserves further detail here. Homocysteine at high levels is perhaps the most inflammatory chemical in the body and relates to brain atrophy,[326] cognitive decline,[327] and coronary vascular disease.[328] It also increases the risk of stroke.[329] Homocysteine is a normal byproduct of amino acid metabolism, but it becomes elevated, and therefore dangerous, when the body does not break it down and recycle it. This happens when a deficiency of vitamins B6, B12 or folic acid are present; making these substances two important hormetic nutrients for balancing Heart 1. Blood sugar problems,[330] liver dysfunction,[331] estrogen creams, and even birth control pills,[332] can cause deficiencies of these nutrients.

The vitamins B6, B12, and folic acid do their work breaking down homocysteine within a cyclical set of steps, known as the methylation pathway. Details of this pathway were discussed in the chapter, *The Fountain of Youth & Anti-Aging?*

Red people, as discussed in *What Color Are You?* are the ones most at risk for elevated homocysteine levels and are therefore at much greater risk for a heart attack. Wheat products ingested by Red people tend to strip them of the vitamins B12, folic acid, and B6, setting them up for homocysteine overload.

Chapter Highlights

- The neurotransmitter norepinephrine directly relates to the PEP Heart 1 and increases with the presence of the fight-or-flight response.

- The heart, a muscle, has the same mineral requirements as all muscles. Imbalances or deficiencies within the necessary minerals, such as calcium, magnesium, potassium, and even sodium, will lead to heart beat irregularities and high or low blood pressure.

- High blood pressure has many causes that patients can manage quite nicely with a functional approach rather than a pharmaceutical one.

- Hypertension is one of the most common reasons for placing a patient on pharmaceutical medications.

- Homocysteine is an amino acid produced in all people. If the body does not detoxify it properly, it becomes one of the most inflammatory chemicals in the body and directly relates to an increased risk of heart attack.

- Low blood pressure corresponds to mineral needs and a deficiency of an adrenal gland hormone called adrenalin.

- Cholesterol and heart attacks do not have a direct relationship. See the chapter *Fueled or Fatty?* for a detailed discussion of the topic.

- The methylation pathways are a primary concern for those with high homocysteine levels and have become a focused area of study for researchers looking for answers to genetic diseases.

TIRED OR STRESSED? – TRIPLE WARMER 23

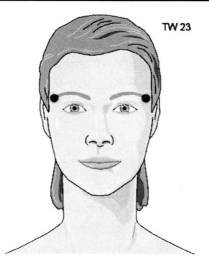

Figure 20: Triple Warmer 23

Related Neurotransmitter: Aspartate, Glutamate (low levels)

Organ or System: Thyroid and Adrenal Glands

Main Biomarkers: Adrenaline, Cortisol, TSH, T4, T3

Common Hormetic Nutrients: Copper, L-Tyrosine, Pantothenic Acid (B5), Potassium, Iodine, Magnesium, Ashwagandha

The PEP Triple Warmer 23 (TW 23) directly relates to two hormone-producing tissues, both related to energy and stress management: the thyroid and the adrenal glands. Both of these can become overworked and eventually fatigued due to blood sugar imbalances, which are the result of a poor diet and emotional stress.

A groundbreaking book by Dr. Datis Kharrazian entitled *Why Do I Still Have Thyroid Symptoms When my Lab Tests Are Normal?* may be destined to change how the medical world views and treats thyroid cases. In it, Dr. Kharrazian states,

The most important thing to remember about the thyroid is that it is highly sensitive to the slightest alteration in the body. It has to be, that's its job. So when the thyroid malfunctions, as it eventually does for an estimated 27 million Americans,[333] the question is not "How can I get 'er up and running as quickly as possible?" but rather "Why on earth is my thyroid mashing the brakes with both feet and yanking on the emergency brake at the same time?"

The chapter *Hypoglycemia or Histamine?* discussed the frequent ingestion of refined foods, sugars, and bad oils and its connection to epidemics of hypoglycemia, insulin resistance, and Metabolic Syndrome. These states, in turn, place great burdens on every other system of the body beginning with the adrenal glands and the thyroid. The initial symptoms generated by these strained tissues include fatigue, insomnia, low sex drive, irritability, and depression. Things, however, often get much worse. Chronic fatigue and fibromyalgia directly relate to TW 23, located at the outer edge of the eyebrows, as well as to other PEPs.

A somewhat paradoxical situation is also common with thyroid and adrenal gland issues. In it, people reach a state of being wired but tired. Those who find themselves in this state may endure fatigue throughout the day, followed by an energy spike at night. Others could experience intermittent daytime panic attacks or heart palpitations just after lying down in bed. All these are signs that tired glands are working to perform vital functions but can only do so in an incongruent and disharmonious way. Like a two-stroke engine sputtering through a bad mix of gas and oil, overworked adrenal and thyroid glands do the best they can with the resources available, which, after years of running a stress marathon, may be paltry at best.

THE THYROID GLAND

The thyroid gland, located behind and adjacent to the 'Adam's Apple' in the throat, is one of the largest endocrine, or hormone-producing glands in the body. Through its hormones, principally triiodothyronine (T3) and thyroxine (T4), it is responsible for important functions, such as energy management and metabolism. The thyroid gland only makes hormones when the pituitary gland tells it to do so. For instance, when the pituitary detects that circulating thyroid hormone levels are running low, it sends out a messenger to instruct the thyroid to get busy. When the messenger, called thyroid stimulating hormone (TSH) arrives, the thyroid gland gets to work making T4. This is step one. Step two is to convert T4, a relatively inactive or weak hormone, into T3. Although it is only seven percent of the total level of all thyroid hormones, T3 is up to 10 times more potent than T4.[334] Sufficient levels of T3 are therefore critical for ample life energy.

When the thyroid becomes out of balance, it will either become too active (hyper) or too sluggish (hypo). Hyperthyroidism is a dangerous situation. Natural means may be able to subdue it, but it often requires traditional medical intervention. Hypothyroidism, on the other hand, is a condition that doctors have misunderstood and therefore misdiagnosed, resulting in millions of unnecessary prescriptions for thyroid medications.

Thyroid imbalance is often a secondary problem. The same disruptors of thyroid function are also the genesis of most functional illnesses. Insulin resistance, immune system dysfunction, hormonal imbalances, [335] and inflammation from food allergies and other gut problems all impede the function of the thyroid.[336] For example, the thyroid gland does not adequately utilize T3 when estrogen levels are too high and may use too much T3 if testosterone levels are elevated. This phenomenon can be observed through a thyroid blood test called, T3 uptake. Insulin, likewise, decreases the sensitivity of thyroid receptors, forcing the body to make more thyroid hormone to produce the same metabolic response. Balancing the thyroid and other primary issues is essential for health and to prevent the onset of an even more ominous condition, thyroid autoimmunity.

AUTOIMMUNE THYROID

One of the scariest, and now one of the most common concerns with thyroid dysfunction, is when the body begins to attack its own thyroid tissue. In the United States, the most common cause of hypothyroidism after the age of six years old is autoimmune thyroid disease, called Hashimoto's.[337] [338] Like all autoimmune diseases, Hashimoto's has a strong connection to females who experience estrogen dominance, polycystic ovarian syndrome (PCOS),[339] those with Celiac Disease, and even those with dental amalgams (mercury fillings).[340] In the case of PCOS, a study reported in the European Journal of Endocrinology 2004, showed that 42.3 percent of women with PCOS had evidence of autoimmune thyroid disease as detected by ultrasound. Despite the fact that Hashimoto's is the primary cause of hypothyroidism and the blood test is inexpensive, almost no one diagnosed with hypothyroidism is screened to see whether they have antibodies against their own thyroid tissue, which is clear-cut diagnostic evidence of Hashimoto's.

Even if doctors do detect Hashimoto's, there is little traditional medicine can do. The treatment of choice is a thyroid medication, usually Synthroid. This does nothing to stop the disease; it just supplies the hormones that a broken thyroid no longer can. For those seeking to do all they can to save their thyroid, this approach is greatly insufficient. The body is not merely a bunch of parts. The thyroid is an important component of the endocrine system, which is the complex organization of tissues that make and regulate hormones. When the thyroid fails, it places great stress upon all the hormone producing tissues of the body such as: the pituitary gland, the adrenal glands, the pancreas, and the ovaries. But it gets worse.

Besides the expected symptoms of low thyroid function, such as fatigue, weight gain, morning headaches, depression, constipation, and so forth, autoimmune thyroid patients often suffer from both hyper and hypothyroid symptoms. When the immune system is actively destroying thyroid tissue, it releases excessive amounts of thyroid hormones. This destruction is what initiates the hyperthyroid symptoms, such as heart palpitations; inward trembling; increased pulse rate, even at rest; insomnia; night sweats; and feeling nervous or emotional. Then, when the immune system is more inactive, hypothyroid symptoms are present.

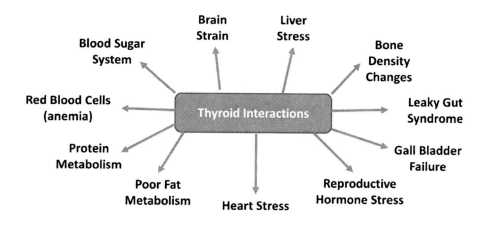

Figure 21: Thyroid Interactions

Blood tests for Hashimoto's include thyroid peroxidase antibodies (TPO) and anti-thyroglobulin antibodies.[341] But just getting thyroid antibodies tested may be incomplete. Autoimmunity begets autoimmunity. 12 percent of Hashimoto's patients also have pernicious anemia, another autoimmune disease wherein the body attacks a substance called intrinsic factor, which is necessary for the absorption of vitamin B12.

Autoimmune disease is a frightening situation. The longer it stays active, the worse it becomes, and the more likely it is that another autoimmune disease will manifest. The key to managing any autoimmune problem, including Hashimoto's, is to leave no stone unturned. Every cell in the body has thyroid hormone receptors. The more thyroid function is disrupted, the greater the chance for a complete functional breakdown. Given the delicate balance of the immune system, any potential cause that may tip the scales is worthy of consideration. In the experience of many complementary medicine doctors, Hashimoto's has a strong correlation with persistent viral infections,[342] heavy metal toxicity,[343] and gluten intolerance. [344] [345] [346] Other practitioners find that deep-seated emotional stressors and continuous exposure to electromagnetic fields are potential triggers for autoimmune flare-ups. Be sure to read the chapter *Infection or Autoimmunity?* for more details on this subject.

In a normal thyroid situation, synthesized T3 and T4 as well as the amino acid L-tyrosine, often offer very good support for the thyroid gland, with one big exception. If Hashimoto's is present, iodine, because it stimulates thyroid function, will make matters worse. Synthesized T3 and T4 utilize iodine. In the short run, patients with fatigued thyroid glands may feel better taking iodine. This is only because their immune system is now aggressively destroying thyroid tissue, causing a temporary release of additional T4 and T3. Continued ingestion of iodine supplementation means these patients will soon crash and burn.[347] The good news is that with FBA, a strong muscle will become weak in the presence of a substance that over-stimulates the immune system. Therefore, practitioners can rapidly screen for iodine or any other suspicious agents.

Thyroid Hormetic Nutrients

Like any hormone, the body must make T4 and T3, utilize them, and finally break them down. Different hormetic nutrients work to support each of these steps. Thyroid health is dependent upon minerals, such as zinc and selenium. Production of thyroid hormones requires iodine and the amino acid L-tyrosine. The thyroid gland also produces a hormone called 'calcitonin,' which plays a role in calcium homeostasis, directing calcium to move into the bones when needed. Thyroid dysfunction of any sort can also disrupt this process, making calcium and magnesium important hormetic nutrients for reestablishing thyroid balance. A person can support and regulate thyroid function during times of stress with the herbs ashwagandha, chasteberry, Peruvian maca and panax ginseng.[348] Finally, if Hashimoto's is present, immune system modulation becomes critical. Vitamin D,[349] omega 3 essential fatty acids, and powerful antioxidants, such as glutathione, are then essential.

THE ADRENAL GLANDS

One adrenal gland sits atop each kidney. Working in concert, the adrenal glands steadily pump out hormones vital for a host of functions, including the following ones:

- Blood sugar balance
- Stress management
- Metabolism
- Immune system regulation
- Proper sleep patterns
- Mood stability
- Musculoskeletal tone

There are three classes of hormones secreted by the adrenal glands: the glucocorticoids, catecholamines, and mineralocorticoids. Any or all of these three classes of adrenal gland hormones can be out of balance when a functional illness is present.

The glucocorticoids – The adrenal glands produce these in response to stressors, such as emotional upheaval, exercise, surgery, illness, or fasting. The most recognizable of the glucocorticoids is cortisol, discussed later in detail.

The catecholamines – These serve as hormones or as neurotransmitters and include such compounds as epinephrine (adrenaline), norepinephrine, and dopamine. The medulla, the inner part of the adrenal gland, secretes epinephrine and norepinephrine, which are the main substances related to the fight-or-flight response.

Mineralocorticoids – These are hormones with specific tasks related to minerals. Aldosterone, for instance, directs the kidneys to retain sodium in times of dehydration.

Acting as the peacemakers of the hormonal family, the adrenal glands will exhaust all diplomatic options while attempting to maintain metabolic order. In the end, their ongoing sacrifice often initiates and then perpetuates vicious cycles that are destructive to the entire endocrine system, while leaving the glands themselves run-down and needing the most attention.

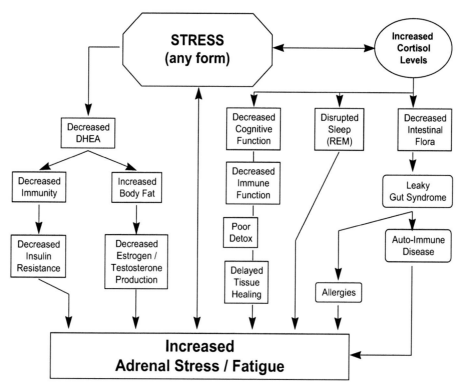

Figure 22: The Stress Effect

To measure the extent of the damage caused by the stresses of life, researchers have designed laboratory tests using saliva to detect and calculate specific adrenal hormones, with cortisol being the most important one.

Cortisol, which is manufactured in the outer part, or cortex, of the adrenal gland, is a multi-purpose steroid hormone that has anti-viral, anti-bacterial, and anti-inflammatory properties.[350] [351] It is also a critical agent involved in blood sugar stabilization, mood balance, and restful sleep.[352]

However, chronic elevations of cortisol, like what occurs with ongoing stress, eventually suppresses the action of the immune system, thereby increasing one's chances for infection. High cortisol will also lead to weight gain by promoting fat storage and muscle tissue breakdown, a process called catabolism.[353] Two diseases relate specifically to cortisol. Cushing's syndrome is the chronic over-production of cortisol, where Addison's disease is just the opposite. Both diseases are rare when compared to the functional imbalances altered cortisol levels create, which are epidemic.

The Circadian Cortisol Profile is a saliva test measuring the normal rhythm of cortisol through a 24-hour period. A normal profile is shown below.

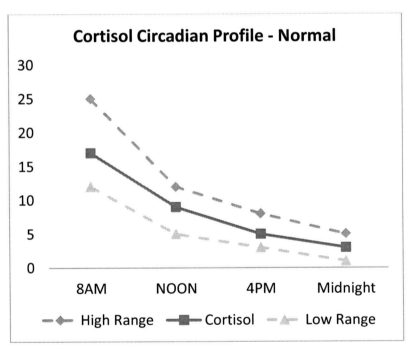

Figure 23: Normal Adrenal Function

The normal rhythm for cortisol begins with high levels in the morning, followed by decreasing levels throughout the day, and ends with the lowest level at night. In the early stages, functional imbalances generated via diet, lifestyle, or other stressful circumstances, begin to alter the flow of cortisol. Eventually, the normal rhythm gets flipped on its head.

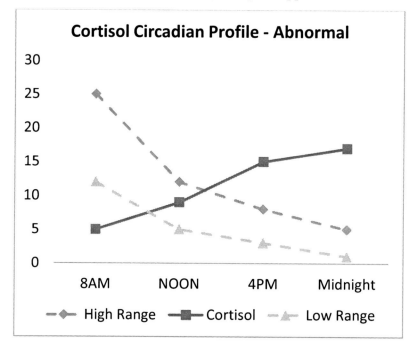

Figure 24: Overworked Adrenal Glands

Elevated cortisol levels at night begin to disrupt sleep and make "popping out of bed" in the morning more difficult. In addition, those with the profile above will likely experience sugar cravings and, if they are female, hormonal swings during their menstrual cycle.

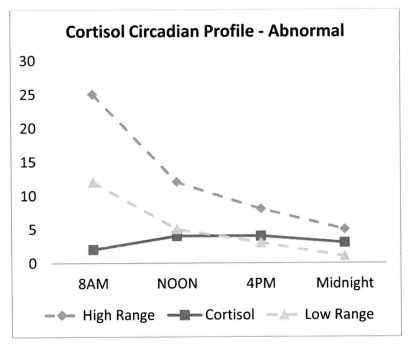

Figure 25: Exhausted Adrenal Glands

The final profile above is adrenal gland exhaustion. It shows cortisol at very low levels, lacking the ability to spike at all. Restoring health in this individual would take time and precision. An all-in-one adrenal gland supplement would not do and might, in fact, further overwork the gland. With FBA, practitioners can discover the ideal hormetic nutrient and supply it in a non-stressful dosage.

Adrenal Gland Hormetic nutrients

Many hormetic nutrients may help restore adrenal function because of their multi-purpose nature and because different degrees of adrenal fatigue are possible. Common nutrients include phosphatidyl serine; vitamins B5, B1, and B2; glandular tissues or extracts; the amino acid L-tyrosine; and calcium or magnesium. In more severe cases, patients may need to supplement adrenal hormones. Bovine adrenal tissue or their extracts can be helpful, as well as hormones such as DHEA or progesterone. Modulating herbs like ashwagandha, rhodiola, and panax ginseng can also be of great value.

Chapter Highlights

- TW 23 relates to the thyroid and adrenal glands. Factors, such as blood sugar imbalances, poor digestion, and systemic inflammation, can push these two tissues out of balance.

- FBA can evaluate these organs with the biomarkers cortisol, adrenaline, noradrenaline, TSH, T4, and T3, as well as many others.

- The thyroid gland is essential for energy production and metabolism.

- Autoimmune thyroid disease, called Hashimoto's, is now the most common form of hypothyroidism.

- The adrenal glands are the stress glands, helping manage stress by releasing hormones, such as cortisol, aldosterone, and adrenaline.

- Saliva tests can effectively manage the adrenal gland hormones and determine the overall level of fatigue for the glands.

ALLERGIES OR INFLAMMATION? – SMALL INTESTINE 19

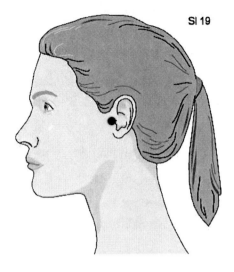

SI 19

Figure 23: Small Intestine 19

Related Neurotransmitter: Norepinephrine (low levels)

Organ or System: Small Intestine

Main Biomarkers: Foods, Fats, Food Additives

Common Hormetic Nutrients: L-Glutamine, Digestive Enzymes, Morinda Citrifolia, Probiotics (acidophilus)

It has been the operating hypothesis throughout *Hope for Health* that functional illness begins with the mouth, which is the first part of the digestive system. A processed and highly refined food diet and the demands it places on the small intestine are the principle reasons why this is so. Located in the middle of the digestive tract, between the stomach and the large intestine, the small intestine is a 30-foot long organ where the majority of food absorption takes place. Enzymes, acids, and good bacteria all work together to break down fats, proteins, and carbohydrates into their smallest parts. The body then uses these raw materials for fuel and for the growth and repair of all cells and systems. Because this is where the yeoman's work of digestion occurs, the body keeps a watchful eye on the entire process via the immune system.

The small intestine contains up to 70 percent of the immune system cells and tissues. Any disruption of the integrity of its linings can lead to inflammation, allergies, and digestive issues of all kinds. This fact is what makes the small intestine a major player in functional illness. And it is why the primary energetic point SI 19 is commonly found at the top of the hierarchy with FBA.

Whenever the immune system does its work of fighting off infections or cleaning up cellular debris, the result is always some level of inflammation. In a healthy immune system, the levels of inflammation go undetected and unnoticed in daily life. This isn't the case when the immune system becomes unbalanced. In this state, a forest fire of pain and swelling can erupt. When inflammation is high in the digestive tract, a host of undesirable consequences emerge, the worst of which is a condition known as Leaky Gut Syndrome.

LEAKY GUT SYNDROME

Decades of ingesting refined sugars, bad fats, and processed foods—the 'sweets and grease' of the Standard American Diet—will inevitably lead to functional problems of all kinds. The lining of the small intestine simply cannot withstand this toxic barrage indefinitely. With every bite of processed food, the immune system increases its activity, ramping up its output of macrophages, phagocytes, and eosinophils, which are the cells responsible for cleaning up the mess. As the response increases, it challenges the stability of the small intestine. Ultimately, the lining transforms for the worse. What was once a tightly knit cellular wall allowing only selected items to move past, now contains gaping holes through which entire proteins pass directly into the blood stream.

Proteins leaking, or translocating, into the blood stream cause a further burst of immune system activity. Antibodies form and attach themselves indiscriminately to everything that comes down the pipe. This means that people with a leaky gut are often allergic to a majority of what they eat. Even the simplest foods, like brown rice and green vegetables, can cause severe bloating and abdominal pain.

Leaky Gut Syndrome is the slippery slope of functional illness. If left unattended, digestive trouble will soon spill over, causing strain on the liver, kidneys, and bladder. These are the detoxification organs responsible for cleaning up the waste products of digestion. With an inflamed small intestine, they must now work around the clock to eliminate the massive load of chemical waste products produced by the restless immune system, creating a state of autointoxication. Signs of poor detoxification will always manifest in those with an inflamed digestive tract. Allergies, chemical sensitivities, digestive complaints of all kinds, headaches, brain fog, memory loss, and fatigue are all common.

Long before the gut can become leaky, a natural barrier must first be overcome. The microflora, or flora for short, is the name for all the good bacteria of the intestines. Up to 700 kinds of organisms make up the approximately five pounds worth of floral material. Acting as a semi-organ, the flora is responsible for helping the body make certain B vitamins and for assisting the immune system by keeping parasites, bad bacteria, and yeast in check. However, this first line of defense has vulnerabilities.

Antibiotics, alcohol, caffeine, food preservatives and additives, and infections from other foods and beverages will all lead to changes in the gut flora. Other chemicals, such as birth control pills and prescription or over-the-counter pain medications add further insult to injury. When ratios of good to bad bacteria become altered significantly, the flora enters a state called dysbiosis. If not addressed quickly, Leaky Gut Syndrome will soon follow.

Chemicals, both from normal metabolic processes and from the diet, create free radicals through oxidation. As explained in the chapter, *The*

Fountain of Youth & Anti-Aging, this constant bombardment drains the body of the important antioxidant glutathione. Once its levels are depleted the tissue-destroying agent iNOS runs rampant. Its presence is directly related to Leaky Gut Syndrome and autoimmune disease.

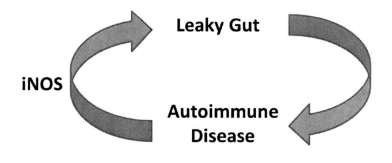

Figure 24: Vicious Cycle of iNOS

From the standpoint of hormetic nutrients, Leaky Gut Syndrome often leads to several mineral deficiencies, including magnesium, zinc, copper, calcium, boron, silicon, and manganese. Even if these minerals are high in the diet, they may not be getting to their target tissues. The inflamed linings of the small intestine disrupt the normal attachment of a mineral to its carrier protein - the taxi that drives the mineral to the cell hotel. Abandoned minerals never make it out of the gut. Fibromyalgia patients, those with chronic whole-body pain and fatigue, consistently demonstrate low red blood cell magnesium even with high magnesium consumption through diet and supplementation.

Once the gut becomes leaky, just taking deficient minerals will not be enough to help. The gut wall must first be healed. Herbs such as slippery elm bark,[354] marshmallow root[355] and deglycyrrhizinated licorice[356] gently repair the mucosal linings of the small intestine.

Functional medicine doctors believe a healthy gut equals a healthy person. They are right. Without a healthy digestive system, overcoming chronic illness is simply not possible. So, proper nutrition is critical.

However, all the best nutraceuticals in the world will do nothing to correct Leaky Gut Syndrome if the diet is not changed.

A diet designed to heal Leaky Gut Syndrome would be free of processed and preservative-filled foods, which would protect the gut from dysbiosis. To prevent blood sugar spikes and insulin surges, it would be low in sweet foods and be protein-based. It would be absent of gluten and most other grains, which would prevent autoimmune reactions. To reduce cellular inflammation, it would contain plenty of natural unheated oils. Finally, it would be full of a variety of colored foods to increase antioxidant activity.

FOOD ALLERGIES

As mentioned above, an overactive immune system will target whatever passes by. This includes food. Food allergies in civilized countries are increasing at a steady rate. In 2007, around three million children had allergic reactions to food. This number represents an 18 percent increase in just a decade.[357] Wondering why this is so, researchers are rightly looking to the flora for answers. Not surprisingly, big differences are present in the flora of those with or without food allergies.[358] However, the flora is just one piece, albeit an important one, of a much bigger functional picture.

Diet determines flora. The bacteria composition of those who eat a diet of mostly vegetables and whole grains will look much different than the flora of those who eat a plethora of refined and processed foods. In the latter case, the gut environment is an ideal place for inflammation and food allergies to spawn.

Food allergies can range in severity from a gas-producing nuisance to a life-threatening anaphylactic reaction.[359] No matter the intensity, food allergies always elicit an inflammatory response. The continuous ingestion of foods strenuous to the digestive tract leads to a hypersensitive immune system. Hypersensitivity is a dangerous thing. Doctors can find the symptoms of it in those who swell, itch, and break out in hives for "no apparent reason." In time, these temporary discomforts will likely mature into something much worse. In many cases, arthritis, for instance, directly relates to food allergies, a phenomenon studied for more than 50 years.[360] The foods most associated with arthritis include the following things: corn, wheat, pork, oranges, milk, eggs, beef, and coffee.[361] Scarier still are the autoimmune diseases that are emerging in epidemic-like proportions. This topic is discussed in the chapter *Infection or Autoimmunity?*

FOOD SENSITIVITIES

From a functional illness perspective, a true food allergy need not be present in order for foods to cause damage. Many people suffer from food-related ailments even though blood analysis does not reveal antibodies, which define a true allergy. Foods can become troublesome simply by eating the same thing too often. There is no such thing as a perfect food. This means the body will need to use some degree of resources in the form of hormetic nutrients to process and eliminate food. This is true for the good foods as well, such as spinach and broccoli.

Healthy foods often have high levels of specific nutrients, like iron in spinach for example. This may sound good at first. However, in a patient low in zinc or copper, excess iron would be detrimental. FBA practitioners have reported that mysterious joint pains, nose bleeds, uterine cramping, and headaches have all abated simply by having the patient stop eating spinach. This, of course, does not mean that people should remove spinach from the dinner table. It simply illustrates that people need to use wisdom in all things. It also indicates that the food proverbs of the past are safe to challenge. What is good for one may be harmful to another.

TREATING ALLERGIES AND SENSITIVITIES

The immune system generates all the symptoms associated with an allergy or sensitivity. If these reactions were slowed or halted, the symptoms would necessarily abate. Treating allergies and sensitivities is possible in impressive fashion via natural techniques designed to override the typical allergic response. N.A.E.T.,[362] BioSet,[363] Acupuncture,[364] laser therapy, specialized chiropractic procedures,[365] and certain forms of energy balancing[366] are all viable options based essentially on the same fundamental idea.

Step 1 is to expose the patient to the allergen itself in order to initiate a mild immune response. The safest way to do this is either to have the patient hold the offending substance in his hand or to simply place it on the body as the person reclines in a relaxed position. This method prevents any potential extreme reactions or anaphylaxis that could occur if the individual tasted or smelled the substance. The proximity of the substance is more than enough stimulation via the electromagnetic matrix for recognition by the nervous and immune systems (see the section *Everything is Electromagnetic* for more details). Once the body detects the substance, the immune system takes action, but the reaction is in a much milder than if the person ingested the substance. It is this low level response that makes Step 2 possible.

Step 2 is to override the immune response with another, more powerful stimulation. This action desensitizes the immune system to the substance. What is important is that the new stimuli be greater than the irritation of the allergic substance and, just as importantly, that the stimuli focuses on organs or tissues related to the immune system. Just adhering to these rules has resulted in remarkable success with natural allergy treatments. FBA can do even better.

The more precise a treatment can be, the better the overall outcome. A sensitive or allergic food will generally cause a strong muscle to weaken if it is on or near the body. When the test muscle weakens, the FBA practitioner can search for the PEP that restores strength. The energetic point that manifests is unique to the patient; it is not likely to be the same for everyone, even if they have the same allergy. Each body reveals which energetic point will do the most good counteracting the allergen. Not surprisingly, paying attention to the specific requirements of the body provides superior results when compared to those with a one-size-fits-all approach.

The anecdotal and laboratory evidence for the effectiveness of natural allergy elimination is abundant. So much so, that many books cover the topic and natural clinics that specialize exclusively in allergies have been opening up everywhere.

Desensitization protocols may be the only hope for relief from allergy symptoms for those with multiple underlying issues. Of course, their effectiveness is greatly enhanced by a holistic approach. A good place to start to produce the best overall result is to do whatever possible to reduce inflammation. Remember, all allergies are inflammatory. Inflammation is like a fire. An influx of water can put out a fire, as can removing the fuel it needs to burn. Stresses of all kinds, like blood sugar and hormonal imbalances, are the fuel. Hormetic nutrients and corrective lifestyle changes are the water. By reducing stress through diet, exercise, and detoxification, people take away the fire's fuel. Doing this at the same time quality nutritional therapy is begun is a sure way to fix the trouble and to prepare the body for allergy elimination techniques.

Chapter Highlights

- The Primary Energetic Point (PEP) most associated with allergies and digestive inflammation is small intestine 19, located immediately in front of the ear canal.

- Allergies begin in the small intestine, which contains up to 70 percent of the immune system.

- Whenever the immune system does its work of fighting off infections or cleaning up cellular debris, the result is always some level of inflammation.

- Chronic intestinal inflammation disrupts the integrity of the linings of the small intestine, making them more porous and "leaky." This creates Leaky Gut Syndrome.

- Protecting against inflammatory assault is one of the jobs of the gut flora, a symbiotic group of over 600 types of microorganisms that live within and are an essential part of the health of the gut.

- Foods directly influence the contents of the flora. Poor food choices lead to poor gut flora and an over active immune system.

- Food allergies and food sensitivities both result from an over-active immune system.

- FBA can correct food allergies and sensitivities by "desensitizing" the body, a process that calms the hyper-immune response.

INFECTION OR AUTOIMMUNITY? – CONCEPTION VESSEL 19

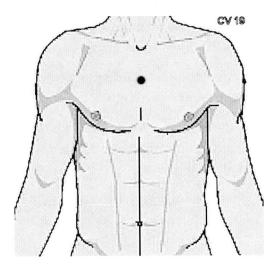

Figure 25: Conception Vessel 19

Related Neurotransmitter: None

Organ or System: Immune System

Main Biomarkers: Immune System Hormones (cytokines)

Common Hormetic Nutrients: Zinc, Vitamin C, Vitamin D, Essential Fatty Acids, Camu Berry, Reishi Mushroom (Ganoderma Lucidum)

Currently, humanity is experiencing the longest life spans since the time of Moses. And yet, the rates of cancer, heart disease, obesity, and diabetes are also at their highest levels. How is it possible that these two facts can be true at the same time? The answer is modern medicine's and modern society's greatest achievement—microbial management – the eradication of bacteria, viruses, and other disease-promoting microorganisms.

Throughout history, invasive microorganisms have plagued society, wiping out thousands, even millions, of people in a very short period of time. Cholera, pneumonia, malaria, Spanish flu and, of course, the Black and Bubonic plagues in total have killed hundreds of millions of people.

In recent history, the Ebola virus and AIDS have scourged the third world and industrial society, respectively.

For the great work accomplished in the areas of disease control, the scientists of medicine and sanitation deserve the praise of all. Because of their achievements in microbial management, plagues are less of a concern today, although scares still remain, as in the recent case of the Asian bird flu. Presently, for civilized society, microbes are less often a threat to life but are a tireless threat to health and to the expression of full human function.

One could make a strong case that bugs, such as bacteria, viruses, fungi, and parasites, are the cause for all disease and dysfunction. Rarely, if ever, will a practitioner find a condition unrelated to bugs to some extent. Heart disease, for instance, is directly linked to burrowing bacteria called helicobacter pylori.[367] [368] The primary cause for hypothyroidism in America is autoimmune thyroid, or Hashimoto's. This process of thyroid self-destruction is many times the result of a virus.[369] Diabetes directly connects to imbalances between the "good" and "bad" bacteria in the digestive tract.[370] [371] Arthritis may in fact relate to a deep-seated infection.[372] Cancer, many believe, results from poor gene expression, which has direct ties to the constant assault of microorganisms, such as the human papilloma virus and its relationship to cervical cancer.[373] Additionally, researchers are investigating the association between breast cancer and three other viruses,[374] one of which is the Epstein-Barr virus, the cause of mononucleosis, a common ailment among teenage girls.[375]

Even if an organism is not directly involved in a disease, its mere presence still requires an immune system response, which results in a continual drain on the body's nutritional resources. Therefore, if people can manage, quarantine, or kill the microorganisms, there is a good chance they can maintain health and extend longevity.

THE IMMUNE SYSTEM

An incredibly complex defensive network, called the immune system, is the body's main form of resistance against various stressors. Up to 70 percent of all immune system cells are in the linings of the intestines. A person's greatest exposure to the outside world is through the food he eats, which may be full of harmful chemicals or bacteria. This, perhaps, is why people with chronic illnesses and weakened immune systems almost always have digestive complaints at the same time.

The immune system is a conglomeration of various cells and tissues designed to prevent foreign substances and organisms from causing damage to the body as a whole. It also works aggressively to promote healing and tissue repair after injury and to eliminate dead cells and improperly developing cells (cancer). The bulk of the immune system, located within the linings of the small and large intestine, is the Gut Associated Lymphoid Tissue (GALT). The linings of the nose, mouth, throat, and lungs contain another web of immune tissues, called the Bronchus Associated Lymphoid Tissue (BALT). Besides these areas, the organs most responsible for immune system support and function are the bone marrow, thymus, spleen, and liver.

The immune system is one of the most intricate and ubiquitous systems within the body. It should then be of no surprise that the immune system is involved anytime someone is suffering from any sort of ongoing issue, such as pain, fatigue, digestive distress, and so on. When the immune system is in trouble and in need of help, the PEP *Conception Vessel 19*, located in the middle of the sternum, becomes active and discoverable with FBA.

White blood cells, called leukocytes, are the cells that increase in number when the body is trying to fight a new (acute) infection. Without white blood cells, resisting infection is not possible. AIDS, for example, is a condition in which these cells are in effect non-existent. There are several types of white blood cells, each with specific immune-related functions: neutrophils, eosinophils, basophils, monocytes, and lymphocytes. For the purpose of a general immune system overview, the focus shall remain on the last type, the lymphocyte, and its role in fighting unwanted antigens and haptens.

Antigens and haptens are any substances that, when present, generate an immune system response. Examples of antigens include bacteria, viruses, and foreign proteins. Haptens are inorganic, or non-living, things consisting of heavy metals, pesticides, chemicals, etc. The chart below demonstrates the basics of what occurs when an antigen or hapten appears in the body.

The first response by the immune system is to "tag," or mark, any undesirable substance for destruction or elimination. This is the job of the antigen-present cells (APC). Next, the APC sends out specific chemical messengers, called cytokines, which call other important "helper" cells to the scene in order to eliminate the antigen.

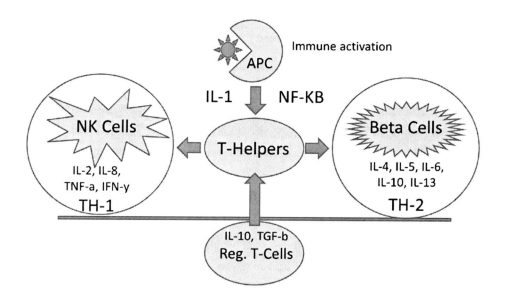

Figure 26: Balanced Immune System

Once the process is underway, the immune system can basically follow two paths, called the TH-1 path or the TH-2 path. The TH-1 path supports the production of natural killer cells (NK cells). The TH-2 path promotes Beta cells. In the early stages of antigen destruction, the immune system relies mostly on NK cells. If the infection is strong or lasts a long time, then it will place more prominence on the production of Beta cells. The Beta cells make people "immune" to things by producing antibodies. For instance, if a person had the chicken pox as a child, she most likely will have chicken pox antibodies in her blood, which ensures that she will no longer get that particular condition. The individual has become immune to the chicken pox.

After the immune system eliminates the antigen, it must turn off the cytokines. Otherwise, there will be a continuous signal for help. There is no need for more wood on the fire when the house is already hot. It is the job of the Regulatory T-cells and the Suppressor T-cells to shut down the immune system when it finishes the job. When all goes well, the antigen is eliminated, cytokines are no longer produced, and the body is now free from invasion/infection. Unfortunately, chronic illness often means the house is either way too hot or it ran out of wood long ago. Either way, the environment is quite uncomfortable.

Before chronic illness sets in, functional imbalances were affecting the body. It is common for the bodies of "normal" or "healthy" people to be in a state of adaptation. Their bodies may have been managing this state for decades. Adaptation simply means the body is using resources from one area to support the deficits of another. Constant adaptation comes at great expense. Eventually, the reserves and tissues responsible for continuing the adaptation process fatigue and finally fail. Like a leaky roof left alone, significant future damage is certain.

Immune system imbalances are no laughing matter. When a dysregulated immune system is present, just about any symptom could result. Worse yet, autoimmune diseases, multiple chemical sensitivities (MCS), Chronic Fatigue, Fibromyalgia, or hypothyroidism, are a long-term likelihood.

For instance, a survey of 1,582 respondents from Atlanta, Georgia found that 12.6 percent reported MCS. The prevalence for this condition is similar in California, where the Department of Health Services reported 15.9 percent, and suggests the national prevalence may be similar.[376] This number is more than double what it was in 2000. In fact, just about all chronic conditions are on the rise and even more so in children.

The number of American children with chronic illnesses has quadrupled in just a generation. According to a study done at Harvard and published in a special edition of the Journal of the American Medical Association on Children's Health, childhood obesity is nearly fourfold in the past three decades and asthma rates have doubled since the 1980s. Likewise, the number of attention deficit disorder cases has skyrocketed.[377] In 1960, only 1.8 percent of American children had a chronic health condition that limited their activities. In 2004, the rate rose to 7 percent.[378]

Because these numbers are steadily going up, it seems logical that immune-compromised and nutritionally deficient people are now giving birth to and raising immune-compromised and nutritionally deficient children. The dietary habits of most children are abominable as well, further perpetuating a worsening state. Unfortunately, the problems don't stop after childhood. They will only get worse.

AUTOIMMUNE DISEASE

Approximately one in five people suffer from autoimmune disease,[379] which is the process whereby one's immune system attacks its own tissues. Autoimmunity is a special threat to women (75 percent), whose prevalence is three times that of men (25 percent). Autoimmune disease is among the 10 leading causes of death for women in all age groups up to 65.[380]

The type of autoimmune disease a person has depends on its location. Rheumatoid Arthritis (RA) affects the joints, Multiple Sclerosis (MS) targets the sheath around the nerves, Type I Diabetes Mellitus affects the pancreas, Crohn's disease attacks the small intestine, and Hashimoto's affects the thyroid gland. These are just a sample of the more than 80 illnesses caused by autoimmunity.

Where Does Autoimmune Disease Come From?

Autoimmune diseases have no precise cause, because they are the result of many causes - a perfect physiological storm. Researchers around the world search for environmental, genetic, hormonal, and nutritional clues without much success. Because all the systems in the body connect, almost any conceivable internal or external cause is possible. Is there still a hidden infection in the gut or mouth? Is the patient full of heavy metals? Has the person eaten foods that the digestive system cannot breakdown or that the liver cannot detoxify? Is there improper genetic expression because of nutritional deficiencies?

No matter what the cause, the cellular mechanisms, those that are out of balance, are becoming clear. These were all described in the chapter, *The Fountain of Youth & Anti-Aging?* Thankfully, PEPs direct the FBA practitioner to those systems that require the most attention. These systems can help the practitioner find the cause of the immune system imbalance. In all cases, to bring the immune system back into balance, certain steps are necessary.

The most common immune dysregulation is an imbalance between the two types of helper cells, TH-1 and TH-2. Often there is an overabundance of immune system activity within one of these categories and not enough with the other. This is yet another of the body's many teeter-totters. Most asthma patients, for example, have a great deal of TH-2 activity, whereas those with Multiple Sclerosis generally have too much TH-1.

When the immune system is teetering, an increase in a group of cytokines, collectively called TH-17, occurs. These chemicals skew the nitric oxide system and dramatically increase iNOS. The result is ongoing tissue damage like what is seen in the autoimmune skin condition psoriasis.[381]

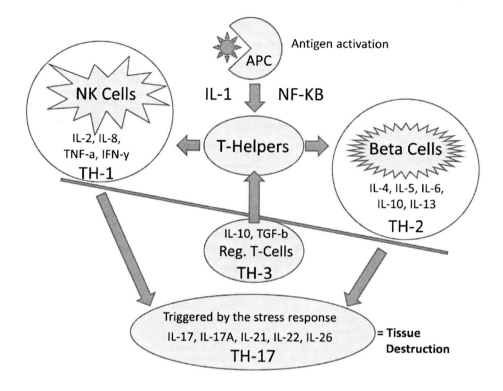

Figure 27: Immune System Out of Balance

The way to regulate this imbalance is threefold. First, the side that is too active needs to be dampened. This often means removing agents that stoke the immune system's fire. Second, the side that is too low needs to be stimulated. This is done with specific nutraceuticals and hormetic nutrients. Finally, the brake in the middle of the teeter-tooter needs to be firmly applied. These are the regulatory cells called TH-3. Immune modulators such as vitamin D, glutathione and healthy oils are the brakes.

The problem is discovering which side of the teeter-totter is high and which is low. For FBA practitioners, this is no dilemma. The person with high TH-1 activity, for instance, will not test well to substances that stimulate that same side, since it is already too high. Vitamin C, Echinacea, and other TH-1 stimulants will weaken a strong muscle on these people. They instead will strengthen to substances that stimulate the lower, or TH-2, side. The opposite scenario would be true for those with excess TH-2 and low TH-1 activity. Here are some of the practical steps to help with immune system regulation:

- TH-1 function too low – increase it with substances like echinacea, zinc, astragulus, and goldenseal.

- TH-2 function too low – increase it with substances like green tea, caffeine, white willow, and grape seed extract.

- TH-1 or TH-2 function too high – detoxify the immune chemicals (cytokines) that continue to signal for help. This is done primarily by supporting the liver.

- Hit the brakes – To stimulate immune modulation via the regulatory cells (TH-3) add Vitamin D, EPA, DHA, and/or glutathione.

Chapter Highlights

- With FBA, Conception Vessel 19, located in the middle of the sternum, is one of the most important PEPs to consider with immune system imbalances.

- One of the greatest advances in medicine was microbial management, which is the ability to exterminate harmful bacteria, viruses, and parasites.

- Many doctors in both the traditional and complementary world of healthcare believe that microorganisms are the cause of most ailments and diseases.

- A large portion of the immune system begins working when signaled to do so by chemical messengers called cytokines. When they are present, the immune system springs into action via a powerful cascading response designed to eliminate microorganisms, neutralize toxins, and repair damaged tissues.

- Approximately one in five people suffer from autoimmune disease, which is the process whereby one's immune system attacks its own tissues.

- Immune system related illness is rising. One theory is that immune-compromised and nutritionally deficient people are now giving birth to and raising immune-compromised and nutritionally deficient children.

- To balance the immune system with FBA, a practitioner must know which side, the TH-1 or TH-2 path, is overactive and supply the hormetic nutrients accordingly.

MIGRAINES, METALS, OR MINERALS? – KIDNEY 27

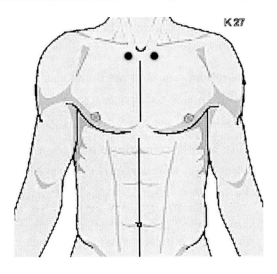

Figure 28: Kidney 27

Related Neurotransmitter: Serotonin (high levels)

Organ or System: Kidneys / Detoxification

Main Biomarkers: Serotonin, 5-HTP, Aldosterone

Common Hormetic Nutrients: Magnesium, Calcium, Vitamin B6, Folic Acid, L-Tryptophan

The kidneys regulate the balance between sodium and water in the body and control the concentration of many other mineral salts, such as potassium, calcium, phosphorus, and magnesium. They also help balance the pH of the body by removing the waste products of physiologic processes. An easy way to support the kidneys is to drink plenty of water—most people suffering from chronic conditions are dehydrated.[382] [383]

The kidneys also produce specific hormones. Renin helps control blood pressure, while erythropoietin is responsible for stimulating the production of red blood cells. The decrease or absence of this hormone inevitably leads to anemia. The activated form of vitamin D, when present in the kidneys, allows the absorption of calcium and phosphorus in the intestine, making the kidneys an essential contributor to bone health. If any of these critical functions begins to fail the PEP K27, located just beneath the collarbones next to the sternum, become active and discoverable by FBA.

MIGRAINE HEADACHES – TOO MUCH SEROTONIN

Migraine headaches affect more than 30 million Americans, including 10 percent of children. According to the National Headache Foundation (NHF), 70 to 80 percent of migraine sufferers have a family history of migraines. A migraine is a severe, debilitating form of headache that typically appears as a throbbing ache near the side of the forehead and can last in some cases up to one week.

There are well-known triggers for migraines and other clues that help define its cause of action and reason for recurrence.

- Women have migraines three times more often than men.[384]

- 75 percent of women get migraines at ovulation or near the start of their cycle.[385]

- Migraines affect up to 37 percent of reproductive-age women, the time when most women are menstruating.[386]

- Common triggers of migraines include noise, light, hormonal changes, sleep disturbances, stress, intensive physical activity, and foods such as chocolate, red wine, cheeses, processed meats, the preservative MSG, caffeine, and alcohol. Food issues often mean trouble with liver detoxification.

From the above facts, it should be easy to recognize that the reproductive hormones (estrogen and progesterone) are somehow a trigger with most migraines. However, other hormones can be involved, as well. Stress, which induces high levels of cortisol and adrenaline, can trigger migraines. So can insulin when released as a result of blood sugar swings. All these issues lead to a suppressed pituitary gland. The section *Balancing Hormones* in the chapter, *Body* Basics, covered the topic of pituitary suppression, but here are a few additional specifics.

The pituitary gland, located about 1 to 2 inches behind the bridge of the nose, is a gland in the body aptly named the master gland. The body cannot secrete hormones unless the pituitary gland tells the body to do so. For instance, if the body needs extra thyroid hormones, the pituitary will send out a hormone called thyroid stimulating hormone (TSH). If the body needs extra adrenal hormones to fight stress, the pituitary will send out a hormone called ACTH to increase cortisol levels. If a woman's progesterone is low, the pituitary sends out luteinizing hormone (LH). If low estrogen is the issue, then out goes follicle stimulating hormone (FSH). This response by the pituitary depends on a negative feedback loop. In other words, when a hormone begins to get low, the pituitary must become activated or facilitated so as to increase the low hormone. When a hormone becomes high, the pituitary must become inactivated or inhibited so the hormone does not become too high (it is the liver's job to eliminate excess hormone).

So, what happens if this very important gland does not properly perform its vital functions because it is either over or under stimulated? This is like driving on the highway with all four tires flat. Since hormones control just about everything, then just about anything symptomatically can occur. For example, if estrogen drops, a suppressed pituitary gland does not respond with FSH. As a result, estrogen will continue to be low. Does the body need more progesterone? This won't happen without LH from the pituitary.

The three most likely pituitary suppressants are insulin, white sugar, and cortisol. The pattern should be growing familiar. Under stress, cortisol increases, causing a person to crave sweets. When ingested (usually in the form of white sugar), the result is the development of hypoglycemia (insulin surges), which can lead to insulin resistance. The vicious combination is self-perpetuating, leading to further pituitary suppression and a massively dysregulated hormonal system. All this is the environment where migraines manifest, but not just yet. Even though hormonal imbalances have a direct link to migraines, the presence of these problems does not mean migraines are a certainty. There is one final factor.

Researchers know that migraines are a vascular headache in nature because of the involvement of blood vessels in the brain. When a chemical trigger is present, the vascular tissues of the brain begin to swell and initiate a migraine. But which chemicals? Perhaps one used by the brain? With FBA, the fuzzy picture becomes clear. The spark that lights the entire hormonal hodgepodge on fire is serotonin.

The chapter *Primary Energetic Points, What to Fix First?* discusses how to navigate the pathways of neurotransmitters. Low or high, as one of the most important neurotransmitters, serotonin makes an impact. When it is too low, it causes depression. Too high results in migraine headaches. The pathway for serotonin is shown below. When too high, it is likely that the necessary hormetic nutrients used to detoxify serotonin are in short supply. FBA can quickly determine this and often yields rapid results, much to the delight of migraine sufferers. Of course, the practitioner will need to evaluate all the other triggers mentioned above, since they are likely to be incendiary.

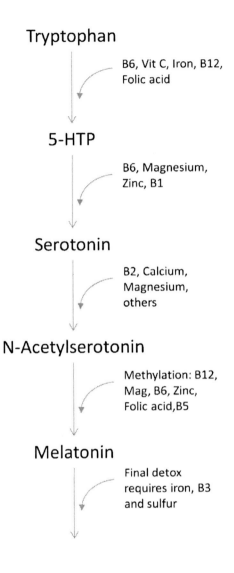

Tryptophan

B6, Vit C, Iron, B12, Folic acid

5-HTP

B6, Magnesium, Zinc, B1

Serotonin

B2, Calcium, Magnesium, others

N-Acetylserotonin

Methylation: B12, Mag, B6, Zinc, Folic acid, B5

Melatonin

Final detox requires iron, B3 and sulfur

Figure 29: The Serotonin Pathway

METAL TOXICITY

Metals of all kinds are a permanent part of the modern conveniences of civilized life, benefit few are willing to forsake. However, as with most things, where there are positives, there are also negatives. Ever since man began working with metal, researchers have found poisonous tendencies. Extensively studied, for instance, are the metals lead, cadmium, mercury, and arsenic. Researchers believe these are the ones that pose the greatest threat to human health. It is now irrefutable that metals cause dysfunction and disease, although debate still rages as to the amount necessary to produce either one. From a functional medicine standpoint, a practitioner must always consider metal toxicity when the PEP K27 becomes active, because the kidneys are the last stage of metal detoxification.

Metal toxicity is a profound disruptor of physiology, often leading to gastrointestinal upset, food intolerances, allergies, vision problems, chronic fatigue, male infertility,[387] and hormonal imbalances of all kinds.[388] But the symptoms do not stop there. Heavy metals inactivate enzymes, the proteins that make everything work in the body.[389] This means that the very things necessary for helping to eliminate metals are themselves turned off by them. Certain metals have an affinity for the nervous system. The brains of Alzheimer's patients often contain a jumbled mass of nerve fibers called a neurofibrillary tangle (NFT). These areas contain high levels of trapped aluminum.[390] Likewise, another degenerative neurological disease, Parkinson's, has a strong association with the presence of mercury and lead.[391]

Where Do Metals Come From?

Metals are everywhere at any given moment. Industrialization has seen to that. People ingest metals regularly through what they eat, drink, and breathe. For those with healthy detoxification pathways in the liver, kidneys, digestive tract, and skin, the body manages and eliminates everyday metals so they do not become a health hazard. Functional imbalances, on the other hand, are notorious detoxification busters and will lead instead to the storage of excess metals. Here is where the problems begin.

When the body has excess metals that it cannot rid itself of, fatty tissue acts like a jailer, trapping the unwanted substances. The more metal that can be "put away," the less total harm to the body. The healthcare industry must recognize this phenomenon of quarantined chemicals before ever beginning a detoxification program. Forcing the body to cleanse itself through a radical, short-term detox will, in some people, do more harm than good. When overweight or obese people lose weight, health benefits abound.[392] [393] However, in the case of cancer, this may not always be true. One study showed that obese people diagnosed with cancer who set out to lose weight and did so to the tune of at least 20 pounds had higher death rates than similar patients who lost no weight.[394] Many in the natural health field believe this seemingly contradictory outcome resulted from a toxic overload created by the dumping of chemicals and metals into the blood stream as the body shed fatty tissue. To prevent this toxic overload, slow and steady is by far the best approach with metal removal.

Most people are aware of the heavy metal mercury and its effects on the body. The general population is primarily exposed to mercury via older dental amalgams and through food, with fish being a major source of methyl mercury exposure. This does not mean fish should be avoided by everyone.

Fish contains good fats that prevent heart disease and protect the nervous system.[395] The Harvard School of Public Health calculated that eating about 2 grams per week of omega-3 fatty acids in fish, equal to about one or two servings of fatty fish a week, reduces the chances of dying from heart disease by more than one-third.[396] However, pregnant women may want to avoid certain fish known to have high mercury concentrations such as shark, swordfish and tuna, since there may be a risk to the unborn baby.

Mercury amalgams are a controversial health topic. Debate over their role as a health hazard and as a cause of various diseases is ongoing.[397] To many in alternative medicine, mercury as a cause of functional illness is undeniable, if for no other reason than the remarkable health benefits witnessed after the old amalgam fillings were removed.

Another metal of concern is cadmium. Society comes into contact with cadmium compounds through re-chargeable nickel-cadmium batteries and cigarette smoke. One reason why cadmium emissions have increased dramatically during the 20th century may be that people rarely recycle cadmium-containing products and often dump them together with household waste.

Lead exposure can occur from drinking water, lead pipes, lead solder, some ceramic dishes, or using lead in hobbies or crafts. Food safety is also of concern. Some meats and spices purchased from foreign countries contain high levels of lead and other metals.[398] [399] The neurotoxic effects of lead have been seen at levels of exposure much lower than previously anticipated.[400] Children, however, face the most serious risk to lead exposure because their growing bodies absorb the metal easily. Lacking a fully developed and protective blood-brain barrier, children's bodies take up the metal into the blood stream, where it then easily travels to the brain. Young children and toddlers play on the ground or the floor and tend to put objects in their mouths. Lead polluted soil, toys covered in lead dust, or in the case of older homes, sweet-tasting lead-paint chips are all possible sources of contamination.

How to Become Metal Toxic without Exposure to Metals

With the teeter-totter effect, an elevated substance means its antagonist is low. In the case of metals, it is always a good idea to look at the high side first, assuming that someone has become metal toxic by excess exposure to the metal. However, all that matters to create health disruptions is that an imbalance is present between the sides of the teeter-totter. This means that that the high side could actually be a normal amount, and the low side could simply be too low. The best example of this idea is the teeter-totter between zinc, iron, and copper, a three-way teeter-totter. The body can rapidly use up each of these three minerals, which are also metals, depending on certain circumstances. Depleted iron results in anemia, depleted zinc results in immune dysfunction, and low copper can contribute to hormonal issues and thyroid problems.

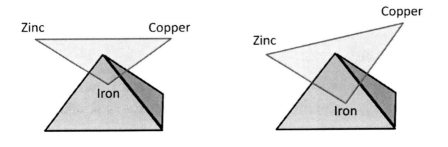

Figure 30: The Copper/Iron/Zinc Teeter-Totter

The picture on the left depicts a three-way teeter-totter with each of the nutrients in proper balance. The picture on the right shows high copper, normal zinc and low iron. Any combination, however, is possible. Each of these nutrients keeps the others in check. In many cases, it activates the function of the others. High iron for instance, will often produce the same symptom as low iron, namely fatigue. Adding the low mineral (copper or zinc) on the teeter-totter will allow the red blood cells to begin utilizing iron once again, and its levels will drop to normal. Why was there a low mineral to begin with? What system, in other words, was using up this mineral too quickly? The primary energetic points (PEPs) will allow the practitioner to find the answers.

Managing Metals with FBA

An FBA practitioner could use a sample of any metal and test a strong muscle to see whether it weakens. However, this is a bit time consuming. Instead, looking for evidence of excess metals is much faster. Because metals have an affinity for the nervous system, neurological deficits emerge when the metals are present in unhealthy amounts. The deficit created by metal overload is easily measured with manual muscle testing via the midline test.

The midline test determines whether the right and left hemispheres of the brain are working synchronously. For example, the left side of the brain controls the muscles on the right side of the body and vice versa. Just lifting the right arm out straight and then returning it to the side is an activity controlled exclusively by the left brain. Now, lifting the right arm out straight and then crossing it over to the left side of the body requires both the left and right sides of the brain to work together. Here is where metals make trouble. They disrupt the normal communication between the right and left brain. Any muscle tested with the arm or leg across the midline will become weak when this communication problem is present.

Of course, the PEPs themselves give the FBA practitioner clues that metals may be bothersome. Often, it is the PEPs most related to detoxification that show up near the top of the list, with Kidney 27 being the predominant one. Finding hormetic nutrients to chelate or attach to metals and remove them from the body is critical. Merely increasing detoxification through hydration is a big help, since it promotes kidney health and function. Furthermore, sweating, a clean diet, and essential hormetic nutrients are all clinically effective.[401]

KIDNEY STONES

Kidney stones may be another indication of a problem with PEP K27. The first signs of a kidney stone appear as pain on the right or left side of the middle part of the back, the thoracolumbar region. The pain, often dull and beginning slowly, soon becomes constant and severe. Other signs may be present with kidney stones, including burning during urination, blood in the urine, or a frequent urge to urinate. With extreme pain, what many describe as akin to labor, nausea and vomiting are also possible.

The shape and appearance of kidney stones depends on which chemicals were responsible for their creation. Most kidney stones are yellow or brown, but they can be tan, gold, or black in color. In shape, they may be round, jagged, or even have a branch-like structure. Kidney stones vary in size. Most are specks like sand, while others are pebbles. In rare cases, stones may be as large as golf balls.

There are five common types of kidney stones. By far, calcium-based stones are the most common. Calcium oxalate stones make up about 70 - 80 percent of all stone types. The remaining types are made of calcium phosphate (often mixed with calcium oxalate), struvite (related to infections), uric acid, and cystine.

Problems and damage resulting from kidney stones may be minimal to severe. The severity of the damage to kidney tissues is dependent upon the location of the stone in the urinary system. To avoid or minimize damage, it is important to eliminate existing stones and, more importantly, to prevent new ones from developing.

Males are four times more likely to develop stones. Other risk factors include family history, chronic dehydration, or little fluid intake. The frequency of stones increases greatly in those with urinary tract blockage, recurring urinary infections, bowel disease, and certain inherited disorders. Because kidney stones are directly related to an inability to properly utilize calcium, any excess calcium in the blood stream can lead to further kidney stones. Even those with no familial history of stones can develop them if blood calcium rises too quickly, as is the case in those who become sedentary due to illness or injury. Astronauts on long space flight are especially at risk since life without gravity immediately begins to weaken bones and dumps calcium into the blood. In these cases, resistance exercises designed to maintain bone density are critical.

The interesting thing about kidney stones is that most sufferers are Blue People. This makes perfect sense. The chapter *What Color Are You?* discusses how Blue people do not fully process dairy calcium. This leads to higher levels of this mineral in the blood stream and the soft tissues, a perfect scenario for future kidney stones. However, doctors rarely advise patients with kidney stones to stop ingesting dairy products. This is a mistake. Instead, doctors may instruct patients to avoid foods containing high oxalate levels, such as spinach. FBA practitioners can easily determine if a patient has high levels of circulating calcium and find the right remedies to normalize this imbalance.

ARTHRITIC OR TOXIC? – LIVER 14

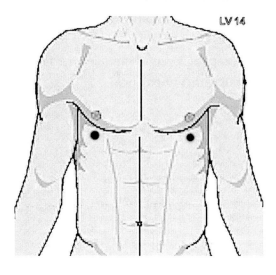

Figure 31: Liver 14

Related Neurotransmitter: Acetylcholine (high levels)

Organ or System: Liver / Detoxification

Main Biomarkers: Acetylcholine, Hormones, Food and Environmental Chemicals.

Common Hormetic Nutrients: Sulfur, Taurine, Iron, Niacin (B3), Magnesium, Milk Thistle, Phyllanthus Fraternus, Schisandra

Think of the liver as a homeschool mom. It cooks (assembles proteins), cleans (converts ammonia to urea), changes diapers (detoxifies), cares for the sick (aids the immune system), makes clothes (produces a variety of essential chemicals), is a counselor (manufactures hormones), takes the kids for a walk (regulates metabolism), monitors behavior (helps regulate blood pressure), saves for the future (stores glycogen and a host of other nutrients), and never sleeps. The liver is responsible for so many functions that it is easy to see why life is impossible without it (her).

The PEP Liver 14 is located on the front of the body just below the nipple. Green people will commonly need their liver supported (see the chapter, *What Color Are You?*), but so do many others. Young women with breast tenderness and cramping during their menstrual cycle are experiencing the effects of liver congestion as it tries unsuccessfully to detoxify the reproductive hormones. Acne is another ailment of adolescence related in part, to an over-worked liver. Liver congestion later in life is the main reason for arthritic pain.

The neurotransmitter imbalance associated with the PEP Liver 14 is elevated acetylcholine. The effect of too much acetylcholine is seen in the muscles of those with the degenerative disease Parkinson's.[402] Acetylcholine forces muscles to contract. As Parkinson's progresses the muscles become more and more rigid. A once normal stride becomes a shuffle and the upper extremities, unable to fully relax, are flexed and unbending.

In the brain, acetylcholine is critical for memory and learning.[403] [404] [405] These desirable effects of acetylcholine would argue that keeping acetylcholine high is a good idea. After all, everyone wants a good memory. However, everything must be in balance. Even too much acetylcholine is not good. Symptoms of acetylcholine irregularities include:

- Decreased visual memory

- Decreased verbal memory

- Slower mental response

- Difficulty calculating numbers

- Changing opinions about oneself

A variety of nutritional compounds can aid the liver in the detoxification process and help lower acetylcholine including: pantothenic acid, thiamin, vitamin C and lithium.[406] [407] [408] Acetylcholine levels, when high, can be made worse with any additional liver stress and even with otherwise beneficial substances such as the amino acid L-carnitine.[409]

HOW DO I BECOME TOXIC?

Today the world is exposed to more chemicals and pollutants than in any previous generation. According to the book, *An Alternative Medicine Definitive Guide to Cancer*, "70 million Americans live in areas that exceed smog standards; most municipal drinking water contains over 700 chemicals, including excessive levels of lead. Some 3,000 chemicals are added to the food supply and as many as 10,000 chemicals, in the form of solvents, emulsifiers, and preservatives, are used in food processing and storage, which can remain in the body for years."

The reason toxins are stored in the body is a matter of efficiency. The human body is a master detoxifier, but everything has its limits. The resources allocated for detoxification are numerous and redundant, but they are still finite. If more toxins come in to the body than can be processed at any given moment, then the body must store them. Storing toxins is much less harmful than allowing them to float freely in the blood. Fat and muscle are typically the storage tissues of choice. Eventually however, if toxin accumulation continues, the immune system suffers and the body then manifests the symptoms of toxicity. Any of the following are possible with toxicity:

Abnormal pregnancy	Kidney dysfunction
Broad mood swings	Learning disorders
Cancer	Memory loss
Chronic fatigue syndrome	Mineral imbalances
Contact dermatitis	Multiple chemical sensitivities
Fatigue	Panic attacks
Fertility problems	Parkinson's disease
Fibromyalgia	Reactions to medications or Supplements
Headaches	Sensitivity to strong smells
Immune system depression	Tinnitus

Foods:

- There are currently 400 different pesticide types available for use.

- 2.5 billion pounds of pesticides are used on croplands, forests, lawns, & fields.

- 24.6 million tons of antibiotics are fed to livestock.

- 750,000 dairy cows are injected with growth hormone.

- Over 80 million acres of genetically engineered crops are presently under cultivation. The long-term effects of these foods are as yet undetermined.

- The average American eats about 125 pounds of additives and 175 pounds of refined sugar per year.

- America leads the world in overall consumption of artificial sweeteners. 800 million pounds or 5.8 pounds of aspartame are consumed per person annually.[410]

Foods with the Highest Concentration of Pesticides	
1. Celery	7. Bell Peppers
2. Peaches	8. Spinach
3. Strawberries	9. Cherries
4. Apples	10. Kale / Collard Greens
5. Blueberries	11. Potatoes
6. Nectarines	12. Grapes (imported)

These statistics have to do with what happens to food before it is prepared to eat. Food preparation - how it is cooked or processed – may also produce toxins. Likewise, food additives such as monosodium glutamate (msg) for some are toxic as well.

Water

The Environmental Protection Agency monitors drinking water for safe levels of microorganisms, disinfectants, disinfectant by-products, inorganic chemicals, organic chemicals, and radionuclides.

- In 2002, approximately 260 million pounds of chemicals were released into surface waters. Since the EPA measures for safe levels and not merely for the presence of toxic substances, you know that the water you consume is already contaminated to some extent. Any water filter is a good idea.

- Many of the pesticides that are eventually dumped into our rivers have estrogenic effects.[411] This means that they act like estrogen hormones in your body, preventing proper hormonal function and production. They also affect the receptor sites where hormones bind,[412] further altering function. It is believed that these estrogenic compounds are responsible in part for the current explosion in hormone cancers, increased hypothyroidism, early female puberty; low sperm counts in males and the loss of libido of both sexes.

- These estrogenic effects take their toll on animals as well. Lake Apopka in Florida, an intensely toxic lake full of pesticides, produced hermaphroditic fish and markedly de-masculinized male alligators. The next generation of alligators born at the lake was 100% female.[413]

- There are also other toxins that are ingested voluntarily such as medications, low quality supplements, birth control pills, recreational and illegal drugs. These too take their toll.

THE LIVER & ARTHRITIS

Arthritis simply means inflammation of the joints: more specifically, the soft tissues that make up the joints such as cartilage and ligaments. Non-autoimmune arthritis, like osteoarthritis, is nearly always associated with an overworked, toxic liver. How the liver becomes toxic is varied, however, food reactions are at the top of the list.

Any food may set off a cascade of chemical events which exaggerate inflammation and encourage the condition of arthritis. So can a host of food additives, preservatives, flavor enhancers and non-food-related substances. Which ones turn out to be trouble makers depends on the genetic and epigenetic variability of a given person.[414] [415] However, some foods are more suspicious than others.

The major inflammers from food are caffeine and its derivatives, gluten (a protein found in wheat and other grains), and solanine, a chemical found in the nightshade family of plants such as tomatoes, potatoes, and spicy peppers. Some people simply do not genetically possess the ability to breakdown certain food items such as alcohol, monosodium glutamate (MSG) and sulfites found in wine and some meats. MSG is a common food additive used as a flavor enhancer but is well known cause of headaches in most Green people (see: *What Color Are You, Red, Green or Blue?*).

Then there are the food toxins. Cheeses for instance, often contain molds. Mold toxins are called mycotoxins and have a direct link to poor DNA replication as well as being a significant stress on the liver. Other foods, like peanut butter, produce aflatoxins, a very poisonous substance believed by some researchers to have a direct link to cancer.[416] [417] [418]

The wrong ratio of good fats and oils will cause inflammatory pain by disrupting eicosanoid balance (see chapter: *The Fountain of Youth?*). Overconsumption of grains or too much of any processed food for that matter, can make life painful as well since nearly all inflammatory reactions begin in the digestive tract.[419] [420]

There are other potential initiators of arthritis including infections and allergies to food additives.[421] Processed meats contain sulphites as do wines. A modest percentage of people have genetic errors preventing the detoxification of sulphites.[422] [423] For these people, synthetic versions of sulfur, such as sulfa drugs, can trigger significant - sometimes anaphylactic - reactions.

Sulfur is the reason why the liver is always involved in joint pain and arthritis. Sulfur is body glue. All soft tissues: joints, ligaments, cartilage, collagen, elastin, and fibrilin, would literally begin to fall apart without sulfur. At the same time, many detoxification pathways in the liver are entirely dependent upon adequate levels of this important nutrient. Ten of the fourteen pathways of phase II liver detoxification are sulfur dependent.

Those with allergies to sulfites or sulfa drugs still need sulfur but lack the ability to utilize all available forms. Sulfur used in detoxification can be free-form or as part of the structure of amino acids such as taurine and cysteine. The liver gets first bids. Whichever available type the liver can use is snatched up, leaving the soft tissue with insufficient amounts of sulfur with which to repair and rebuild.

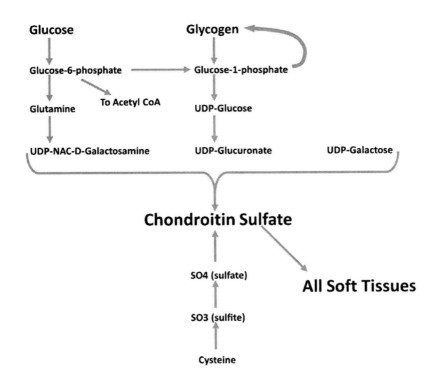

Common joint nutrients available in the local drug store include glucosamine, chondroitin and MSM. These are all different forms of sulfur. But none of these work for everyone. Each body type has its own specific requirements. FBA can determine which one is best in seconds. Above is a review of the formation of chondroitin sulfate, a glycosaminoglycan (GAG) and critical component of many soft tissues. GAGs are like 2X4 studs - the primary building material for the body's soft tissue house.

An important thing to know about GAGs is that they are assembled from sugars (polysaccharides), which cling to an amino acid called serine. It can be seen from the figure above that SO_4 or sulfate is one of three critical precursors to the metabolism of chondroitin (4 or 6) sulfate. The other two are glucose (blood sugar) and glycogen (stored glucose). Each polysaccharide or sugar molecule is derived from glucose via the sugar-using (glycolytic) pathway and connected together to make a GAG.

Just from knowing these three key components it can be theorized that if blood sugar management or liver detoxification were compromised, soft tissue formation and repair would suffer. Poor detoxification often results from a poor diet and is then compounded by a disrupted blood sugar system. The case for liver-based arthritis has now been built.

The pattern goes something like this: A prepubescent female eats the Standard American Diet (SAD) which is full of trans-fats, refined sugars, too many simple carbohydrates, not enough quality protein and a plethora of food additives and flavor enhancers. This diet and other lifestyle factors associated with living in the modern age, place a large strain on the regulation and utilization of both glucose and glycogen. Because the primary fuel for the brain is glucose, the body will do what it must in order to first feed the brain. This means that the sympathetic fight-or-flight system gets turned on in order to generate glucose from muscle catabolism and never gets turned off.

As a result, other blood sugar dependent systems are sacrificed out of necessity as glucose is scavenged to feed the brain - like those that assemble chondroitin sulfate. At the same time, the entire endocrine and glucose system is further stressed by a woman's menstrual cycle. Excess progesterone, estrogen, luteinizing and follicle stimulating hormones require sulfur and a host of other nutrients to detoxify.

The sulfur and nutrient depleted liver is soon overburdened by the hormonal barrage, which results in the recognized symptoms of PMS. This process continues for decades leading to imbalanced hormones, dilapidated joints, scarceness of nutrients and much more.

Chapter Highlights

- Liver disturbances will activate the PEP Liver 14. The neurotransmitter imbalance associated with this PEP is elevated acetylcholine.

- A congested liver means sluggish detoxification. In young women this could mean breast tenderness and cramping during her menstrual cycle. Whereas, liver congestion later in life is the main reason for arthritic pain.

- Tissue toxicity is the result of too much exposure to chemical compounds in the food, water or air supply; from the inability to eliminate toxins effectively, or both.

- Sulfur is both a primary liver detoxifier and a body "glue." All soft tissues: joints, ligaments, cartilage, collagen, elastin, and fibrilin, would literally begin to fall apart without sulfur.

- Continuous liver strain reduces the total level of tissue sulfur, which can then result in osteoarthritis and joint issues of all kinds.

- The hormetic nutrients required most often to support an over-worked liver include: magnesium, sulfur, pantothenic acid, vitamin B12, folic acid, the components of glutathione and herbs like milk thistle and dandelion root.

ADHD OR MISPLACED MEMORY? – CONCEPTION VESSEL 24

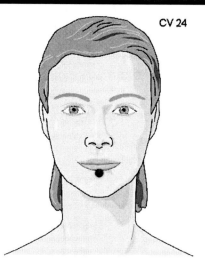

CV 24

Figure 32: Conception Vessel 24

Related Neurotransmitter: Dopamine (low levels)

Organ or System: None

Main Biomarkers: Dopamine, L-Tyrosine, Estrogen (low)

Common Prime Movers: Copper, Pantothenic Acid, B6, Magnesium, L-Tyrosine

Brain health is the body's top priority. As shown in the chapter *The Primary Energetic Points*, the chemicals that modulate mood and behavior in the brain, called neurotransmitters, all directly relate to the PEPs. Consequently, they are discussed in nearly every chapter of *Hope for Health*. Pivoting into a discussion of the brain could therefore naturally spring from any previous page. However, no one is motivated like a parent in search of help for his or her child. Memory, concentration, learning disabilities of all types, and the controversial topic of Attention Deficit Disorder are each associated directly or indirectly to the PEP Conception Vessel 24 (CV 24), making this chapter the best place to segue into a deeper discussion about the brain and its place in functional illness.

CV24 is located in the midline, just below the lower lip. It relates to low levels of the neurotransmitter dopamine. Known as the pleasure neurotransmitter, dopamine accentuates experiences and creates expectations of good things to come. Those with low dopamine levels have low salutogenesis - a term denoting that life can be understood, that it is manageable, and most of all that it is meaningful. The stresses of life easily overwhelm someone with low salutogenesis and increase the potential for functional illness.[424] [425] [426] Low dopamine levels are common in the elderly,[427] among people with Parkinson's disease,[428] and in children prescribed the behavioral drug Ritalin.[429]

ATTENTION DEFICIT / HYPERACTIVITY DISORDER

Attention-Deficit/Hyperactivity Disorder (ADHD) is one of the most common neurobehavioral disorders of childhood, with 5.4 million children diagnosed in the United States alone. That is nearly 1 in 10 school-age children and a million more children than were reported in 2003. Of these cases, 2.7 million are currently taking ADHD medication.[430] Children with ADHD have trouble paying attention and controlling impulsive behaviors. In some cases, they are overly active. Additionally, rates of parent-reported ADHD diagnosis are increasing, and the patterns of ADHD diagnosis are changing.

Typically, a child with ADHD may have the following issues:

- Difficulty paying attention
- Excessive daydreaming
- Trouble focusing on schoolwork or play
- Difficulty staying still or seated
- Excessive fidgeting or squirming

- Trouble talking too much

- Difficulty with playing quietly

- Problems due to acting and speaking without thinking

- Trouble taking turns

- Difficulty listening without interrupting others

What is the cause of ADHD?

Inherited weakness – The number of American children with chronic illnesses has quadrupled in just a generation. In 1960, only 1.8 percent of American children had a chronic health condition that limited their activities. In 2004, the rate rose to 7 percent. Because this number is steadily going up, it seems logical that immune-compromised and nutritionally deficient people are now giving birth to and raising immune-compromised and nutritionally deficient children.

Low nutrient levels – Children with ADHD have low levels of essential fatty acids and do not fully process those they do have.[431] The brain loves oils. Its structure is made up of around 50 percent fats and oils. The chapter *The Fountain of Youth & Anti-Aging* discussed the importance of a proper balance between different types of oils, especially the omega-3 and omega-6 forms. Omega-3 oils from fish contain two important acids for the brain: EPA and DHA. In children with learning difficulties, the DHA portion is often too low.[432] [433] They may also have low levels of zinc,[434] vitamin B6,[435] the amino acid tyrosine,[436] and magnesium.[437] [438]

Food allergies – A critical review of the scientific literature provides very limited support for the idea that food or food additives are a direct cause of ADHD or most functional illness, for that matter.[439] It never will. Traditional medicine only considers food detrimental if it causes a disease like celiac or requires an epinephrine injection to prevent anaphylaxis. A diet of reduced sugar, dairy, wheat, and processed foods has shown to be helpful in studies[440] and repeatedly in the offices of alternative medicine and FBA practitioners.

Immune system reactions – The immune system's ability to destroy joint tissue in the deforming condition Rheumatoid arthritis is well recognized. The immune system can destroy brain tissue, as well. Cytokines are immune chemicals, which circulate throughout the body. When produced excessively in the brain, they can contribute to negative behavioral effects.[441] [442] [443]

Vaccinations – It is undeniable that vaccinations are a potential health risk for some. Vaccine Adverse Events Reporting System (VAERS) details the acute responses reported by parents of vaccinated children, including the following ones:

- Pronounced swelling, redness, heat, or hardness at the site of the injection;
- Body rash or hives;
- Shock or collapse;
- High-pitched screaming or persistent crying for hours;
- Extreme sleepiness or long periods of unresponsiveness;
- High fever (over 103 F);
- Twitching or jerking of the body, arm, leg, or head;
- Crossing of eyes;
- Weakness or paralysis of any part of the body;
- Loss of eye contact or awareness or social withdrawal;
- Loss of ability to roll over, sit up, or stand up; and
- Breathing problems (asthma).

Congress, persuaded by the number and severity of post-vaccination reactions, established the National Childhood Vaccine Injury Act in 1986. Within 10 years, the Federal Vaccine Injury Compensation Program had compensated nearly 1,000 families at a cost of $600 million. Many who speak out against the dangers of vaccinations see a similarity between the rise of ADHD and the ever-increasing number of vaccinations required for children.

The U.S. has one of the highest vaccination rates in the world. The vaccination schedule from the Centers for Disease Control and the American Academy of Pediatrics recommends a child receive nearly 34 doses of 10 different vaccines by the time they enter kindergarten.

Today, there are more than 200 vaccines being created by federal health agencies and drug companies. These include vaccines for Hepatitis C, D and E; Herpes simplex types 1 and 2; gonorrhea; rotavirus (diarrhea); Group A and B streptococcus; meningitis A, B and C; and HIV for AIDS.[444]

The aforementioned reactions and coincidences do not necessarily mean that vaccinations alone are the reason for ADHD. Rarely is any one cause the reason for a functional imbalance or disease. A multi-causal effect is most likely— the proverbial "straw that broke the camel's back" is true in this case. However, multi-causal effects are very difficult to prove in a lab or in a court of law, so the debate, undoubtedly, will continue.

Low dopamine levels – The path that leads to ADHD ultimately ends with low dopamine levels.[445] That is why the PEP CV 24 manifests in most behavioral issues. The ADHD drug Ritalin® assists mood modulation because it enhances the important brain-stabilizing neurotransmitter dopamine.[446] Ideally, from a holistic perspective, rather than augmenting dopamine with a medication, it would be much better to repair the dopamine pathway, thereby correcting several otherwise as yet unrecognized problems simultaneously. The dopamine pathway and some of the important hormetic nutrients needed to make the pathway flow freely are shown below.

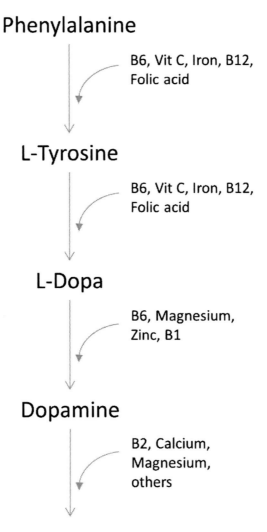

Figure 33: The Dopamine Pathway

MEMORY

According to the Aging, Demographics, and Memory Study, the prevalence of dementia among individuals aged 71 and older was 13.9 percent, comprising about 3.4 million individuals in the USA in 2002. Dementia prevalence increased with age, from 5.0 percent of those aged 71 - 79 years to 37.4 percent of those aged 90 and older.[447]

Concerning dementia, the forms disconcerting for most are related to progressive degenerative diseases like Alzheimer's and Parkinson's. Alzheimer's disease affects almost 10 percent of people over 70 years old, or around 2.4 million individuals.[448] Parkinson's disease affects about 1 million people in the United States.[449] Although the cause of these two diseases is unknown, it is undoubtedly multi-factorial and the result of many health-degrading influences, as discussed throughout *Hope for Health.*

For example, as mentioned in the chapter *Migraines, Metals or Minerals*, the brains of Alzheimer's patients often contain a jumbled mass of nerve fibers called a neurofibrillary tangle (NFT). These areas contain high levels of trapped aluminum.[450] Parkinson's also has a strong association with the presence of mercury and lead.[451] Another strong connection is poor glucose utilization by the brains of dementia patients.[452]

Making matters even more interesting, science has yet to determine exactly which lobes of the brain store memories or whether they store memories at all. The idea that memory is transpersonal (outside the brain) and part of a morphogenetic field, a term that means, "giving birth to form," is an idea that has been around since the 1920s. It is gaining greater traction today. These theories, beyond the scope of *Hope for Health,* are tied to the mysterious world of quantum mechanics. In the years to come, they may garner further consideration.

Making Memories

To make a lasting memory, an event needs one or all of three ingredients: intensity, duration, and repetition. The roots of neurons, called dendrites, make their connections under the modulating influence of dopamine, which brings the discussion back to the PEP CV 24. Acetylcholine, another important neurotransmitter, is important for memory recall.[453] [454]

In order to produce adequate levels of acetylcholine, vitamin B5 or pantothenic acid is required. This vitamin helps choline bind with the important molecule acetyl CoA. Choline can be ingested through food or made by the good bacteria in the gut. Assembling the two parts, acetyl CoA and choline, to make acetylcholine requires the trace mineral manganese, which acts as an "on" switch for a synthesizing enzyme.

FBA can customize the nutrition necessary to enhance memory by determining which of these or other important nutrients are needed most. The other nutrients are most likely related to energy production.

Fatigue often accompanies memory problems. Making, storing, and retrieving memories requires ample amounts of neurotransmitters, which are assembled from an ample supply of amino acids. In the hierarchy of body needs, energy for daily survival is more important than short-term memory. This means that if the body begins to get run down, it will preferentially choose to utilize amino acids for energy creation rather than for making memory-supporting neurotransmitters. The Krebs cycle can steal amino acids to make energy at the expense of memory.

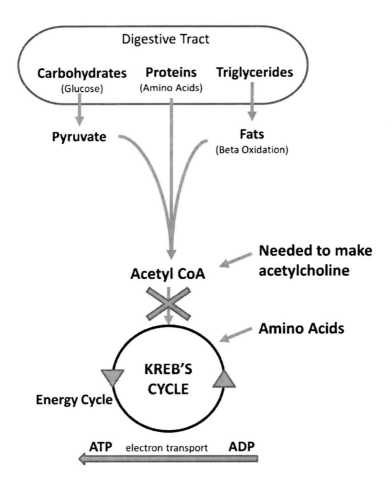

Figure 34: Amino Acids & The Krebs Cycle

The figure above shows how amino acids (like tyrosine, which is used to make dopamine) are stolen by the Krebs cycle in order to provide energy for the whole body. The reason why this aggressive step is necessary is because the important precursor to the energy cycle, acetyl CoA, is no longer getting through. This can happen for a variety of reasons, with insulin surges and other blood sugar system imbalances leading the way.

In the case of memory and all functional imbalances, the whole person approach presents itself as the ideal option. If energy is being lost, one can be sure that more than just memory is suffering. Each of the steps of Functional Bio-Analysis reveals which systems are in the most trouble and the therapies best able to get them out.

BRAIN FOG

Confusion, poor memory, and slow processing are all commonly associated with brain fog. These symptoms are a sign of neurologic fatigue. Different from metabolic fatigue, which occurs after prolonged exercise, neurologic fatigue in the brain is when someone feels tired, or even exhausted, after performing a mental task. Most children with dyslexia, ADHD, or visual or auditory processing disorders experience neurologic fatigue.

From a hormonal perspective, the most common reason for brain fog is thyroid suppression. The thyroid gland is a sensitive tissue that is easily influenced by the hormones and chemicals of other systems, such as elevated cortisol from stress, insulin surges from blood sugar imbalances, and cytokines from the immune system. Other chemicals are provocative, as well. Lipopolysaccharides, the waste products of non-beneficial bacteria in the small and large intestines, are especially toxic to the liver, which in turn affects thyroid hormone production.[455] Basically, brain fog is possible with anything that promotes inflammation or a prolonged immune response.

Brain fog often means that an active inflammatory response is present in the brain itself – it is on fire. The cells of the brain are primarily two types: microglia cells and neurons. Microglia cells are 10 times more numerous than neurons and are the ones most likely to become inflamed. Prolonged brain inflammation will actually degenerate the brain to the point that it shrinks.

To control the inflammatory response in the brain, nutrition must cross the blood-brain barrier or support anti-inflammatory agents that do. Research has shown, and FBA has confirmed, that curcumin,[456] an antioxidant from the spice turmeric; catechin,[457] an antioxidant found in many teas; and some special bioflavonoids called, apigenin, luteolin, and baicalein,[458] [459] [460] can all be helpful.

BRAIN REHAB

It used to be believed that brain function was "fixed" after adolescence and was guaranteed to decline with age. This is not so. The age of the brain is a factor, but to a far lesser degree than how intensely it is used. What is true for muscles is true for the brain and every other organ in the body: "use it or lose it."

The brain is more than capable of modifying, healing, and rewiring itself through the life-long process of neuroplasticity. When stimulated to do so, neurons (nerve cells) in the brain regularly sprout fresh nerve endings to form a new neuronal pathway. This is true with any mental challenge, such as learning a new language or after an injury. For example, if the right side of the brain is damaged as the result of a stroke, the left side may compensate and take over some of its functions. The brain even develops just by thinking about doing something through a process called the mirror neuron system.[461]

Compensation is good in the short term and, in the case of serious injury, may be the best one can hope for. However, to realize the brain's fullest potential, underdeveloped areas need to be exercised. The child who learns to tilt her head in order to read out of her dominant eye may in fact learn to read, but she is also cementing her brain in a compensatory pathway. Instead, she should capitalize on the power of neuroplasticity by strengthening the weak areas through regular use. This will make her whole brain work properly, not just certain parts.

Exercising the brain enhances working memory.[462] The term "working memory" refers to the ability to store and manipulate information to the extent necessary for complex cognitive tasks, such as language comprehension, learning, and reasoning.[463] When working memory improves, so does fluid IQ—the ability to solve problems or adapt to situations as they occur. A greater working memory and fluid IQ are what parents hope to provide their underperforming school-age children.

Memory training takes on many forms and is described by many different names. This is because there are many ways to help a forgetful brain. Memory training for 14 hours over five weeks has been associated with greater dopamine levels in both the prefrontal and parietal portions of the brain.[464] Memory training improves the working memory for all age groups[465] and has the added benefit of making children more aware of their surroundings, more responsible with their school materials, and more aware of social cues. As good as memory training may be, the brain is not simply meant for thinking.

A bulging brain, one that enhances all aspects of life, requires regular stimulation through all the five senses, not just sight and sound. The brain governs all muscle function of the body, making it responsible for movement. The right hemisphere, for example, controls the muscle function on the left side of the body and vice versa. This knowledge is essential for brain rehabilitation. If function is absent or has been lost in the right brain, exclusively using the muscles on the left side of the body will stimulate the right hemisphere and initiate the process of neuroplasticity.

Which Brain Are You?

In the late 1960s, an American physiological psychologist Roger W. Sperry developed the concept of right-brain and left-brain thinking. He was later awarded the Nobel Prize in 1981. The left brain is the detective that studies details. It is logical and sequential, looks at the parts before putting them together as a whole, and is analytical and objective. In contrast, the right brain is the psychic relying on intuition. It is random, looks at the whole before studying the details, and is instinctual, holistic, and subjective.

Most individuals have a distinct preference for one of these styles of thinking. Some, however, are more whole-brained and equally adept at both. In general, schools tend to favor left-brain modes of thinking while downplaying the right-brain ones. This often leaves right-brain learners at a disadvantage. Left-brain scholastic subjects focus on logical thinking, analysis, and accuracy. Right-brained subjects, on the other hand, focus on aesthetics, feeling, and creativity.

To foster a more whole-brained scholastic experience, teachers should use instruction techniques that connect with both sides of the brain. They can increase their classroom's right-brain learning activities by incorporating more pictures, patterns, metaphors, analogies, role-playing, visuals, and movement while working on left-brain subjects. These same ideas can be used to enhance memory.

A Healthy Brain is a Balanced Brain

Some professions thrive because of imbalanced brains. Certain engineers, mathematicians, and scientists are left-brain dominant, whereas some of the world's most renowned artists are overrun by the right brain. To achieve the greatest discoveries and developments, it is probably best to leave both of these groups lopsided. These however, are the exceptions. For the purposes of health and all around wellbeing, most people should strive to have a balanced brain.

The FBA practitioner should have the patient perform a mathematical problem, such as subtracting by threes starting with an arbitrary number like 71. This is a left-brain activity. If a strong muscle goes weak after some simple subtraction, it means that the left brain is too active and the right brain is underactive. Likewise, humming or singing is a right-brain activity. If a strong muscle goes weak after singing or humming "Happy Birthday" for instance, then the right brain is overactive and the left brain is likely to be underactive.

There are a great number of brain exercises available to strengthen the brain. The trick is to know which areas need the most support and which exercises will do the best job. FBA practitioners have a tremendous advantage here. Through manual muscle testing, FBA can analyze both the right and left sides of the brain for deficiencies and find the most effective therapies, as well as the ideal nutrients for brain support. If for example, a patient weakened to a simple subtraction exercise, the practitioner can place nutrients on the body and repeat the exercise. Now, if the patient no longer weakened, then the nutrients are likely to be helpful for balancing the brain.

Using the whole body to balance the brain is critical, as well. If a strong muscle weakens when a patient performs some simple cross-crawl activities on the examining table, it indicates a communication problem between the right and left hemispheres. Cross-crawl is like walking while lying down. While lying face up, a patient should lift one leg off the table while lifting the opposite arm. As the person lowers those parts back to the table, he should lift the opposite leg and arm. Repeating this movement for six cycles should be enough to perform the test. Performing a cross-crawl should not cause a problem in someone with a balanced brain. However, in many people, a strong muscle will weaken.

There are many ways to balance the brain. All sensory information is processed through the brain. This means that all sensory input could potentially help balance the brain. However, some sensory information is processed in the right brain and some is processed in the left. Certain musical notes help balance the right brain and others, the left. Colors do, as well.

Sensory Information Processed in the LEFT Brain			Sensory Information Processed in the RIGHT Brain		
Features	**Colors**	**Sounds**	**Features**	**Colors**	**Sounds**
Math Facts	Red	A	Math Concepts	Green	D
Structured	Orange	B	Colors & Humor	Blue	E
Language	Yellow	C	Pictures	Indigo	F
Short-Term Memory			Long-Term Memory	Violet	G

Table 2: Left & Right Brain Features

Using FBA, a practitioner can find a collection of colors and sounds for use in the office and at home to support balanced brain development. For instance, a right-brain patient already has a highly developed right brain and an underdeveloped left brain. Introducing more right brain stimuli could weaken a strong muscle. These stimuli should be avoided. The patient should be sent home with activities, sounds, and exercises that stimulate left-brain function, such as music in the key of A, B, or C and glasses with the colors red, orange, or yellow. However, a right-brain dominant person will learn and memorize better if right-brain learning styles are used. This means employing pictures, stories, colors, and movement.

Regardless of age or which hemisphere is dominant, the table below lists some simple yet effective at-home brain enhancing ideas that anyone can do.

Brain Builders	
Exercise	Employing cross-body movements and balancing techniques are a great way to make both sides of the brain work as a team. To enhance the effect of daily exercise, cross the midline by swinging the arms across the body while walking. This makes the right and left brain work together.
Balancing	Stand on a balance board while reading or doing dishes. 15 minutes a day.
Switch hands	Do activities with the non-dominant hand, such as brushing your teeth or using the mouse on the computer.
Eyes closed	Use different senses to accomplish the same task. Try getting dressed with the eyes closed.
Break routines	Go to work in a different direction. Stop watching television before bed. Read or solve a puzzle instead.
Play Bingo	Games and puzzles foster concentration and exercise the brain. Bingo has been shown to help keep elderly minds sharp.[466]

PLEASURE OR PARANOIA? – GOVERNING VESSEL 27

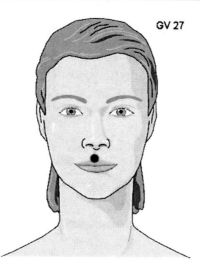

GV 27

Figure 35: Governing Vessel 27

Related Neurotransmitter: Dopamine (high levels)

Organ or System: None

Main Biomarkers: Dopamine, Norepinephrine, Adrenaline

Common Hormetic Nutrients: Copper, B6, B3, Magnesium, Pantothenic Acid (B5)

The PEP Governing Vessel 27 (GV 27) is located at the middle upper portion of the lip at the transition between the skin of the lip and the skin of the face. As discussed in the previous chapter, dopamine is the pleasure neurotransmitter.[467] Too much of this essential neurotransmitter turns pleasure into paranoia. When the PEP GV 27 is active, it means that dopamine levels are high. Symptoms associated with too much dopamine include: feelings of hopelessness, self-destructive thoughts, aggressive tendencies, regular nightmares and restless leg syndrome.[468] Those with elevated dopamine are often easily distracted and find it difficult to complete tasks. In severe cases, high dopamine levels are associated with paranoia, schizophrenia,[469] [470] and even suicidal tendencies.[471]

High Dopamine and Nightmares

Elevated dopamine can result from a defect in the metabolism of the downstream neurotransmitter norepinephrine – the chemical with the greatest influence on the fight-or-flight response. This is the same response that easily disrupts sleep and creates patterns of insomnia. However, once dopamine begins to get involved, insomnia rises to another level. Sleepwalking, nightmares with loud outbursts and violent tossing and turning are common with too much dopamine.[472] These accentuated patterns of disrupted sleep are together called Parasomnias - a category of sleep disorders that involve abnormal and unnatural movements, behaviors, emotions, and perceptions during sleep.

Correcting High Dopamine with FBA

Normalizing dopamine often means trimming back the fight-or-flight response. This topic is covered in detail in the chapters, *Panic or Pass Out* and *Tired or Stressed*. To reiterate, the adrenal gland hormone cortisol is the body's natural antidote and counterweight to norepinephrine, but just increasing cortisol is not enough. Assisting the body in the removal of norepinephrine is essential. Many hormetic nutrients can help. The next step is to lower dopamine.

Any hormetic nutrient listed below could be an important part of lowering dopamine levels. However, people with elevated dopamine often have low nutritional copper. Because of the Teeter-Tooter Effect, this also means that they will have high levels of iron or zinc at the same time. If this if found to be present with FBA, including copper in a person's nutritional regime will aid the metabolism of dopamine while at the same time naturally lower the elevated teeter-totter nutrient (zinc or iron). Patients regularly report significant symptom resolution with this approach. Copper builds up fast in the body so not much is needed. One 2mg pill daily for four to eight weeks is usually sufficient.

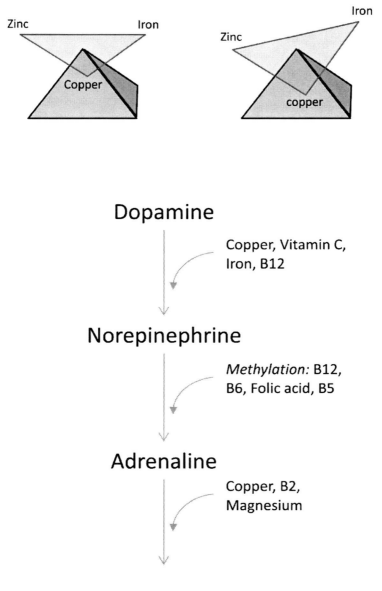

Figure 36: The Dopamine Pathway

ACIDIC, ACNE OR ULCERS? – STOMACH 1

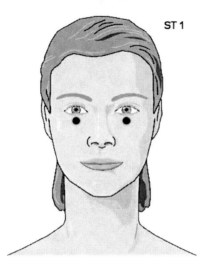

ST 1

Figure 37: Stomach 1

Related Neurotransmitter: Histamine (low levels)

Organ or System: Stomach

Main Biomarkers: Histamine, Histadine, Hydrochloric Acid

Common Hormetic Nutrients: B6, Magnesium, Zinc, B12

The PEP stomach 1 (ST 1) is located just below the bottom of the eye socket, at the apex of the cheeks. ST 1 will show up in the FBA hierarchy and cause a strong muscle to weaken whenever a disruption of the stomach is present, such as duodenal and gastric ulcers, stress gastritis, gastro-esophageal reflux disease (GERD), pancreatic insufficiency, and non-ulcer dyspepsia.[473]

The neurotransmitter related to ST 1 is histamine. This chemical is well known for its ability to cause allergic reactions, such as sniffling, sneezing, and itching. However, when related to ST 1, histamine will actually be low. This means that the immune system is under-functioning.

Oftentimes, if the body has been fighting off an infection for some time but cannot fully eliminate the organism, the immune system will become tired. On a blood test, the leukocytes, or white blood cells, would be below normal. Increasing histamine in this instance would give the immune system a boost.

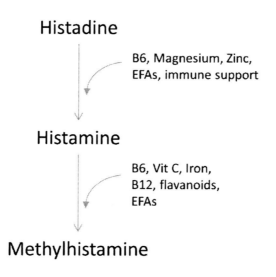

Figure 38: The Histamine Pathway

HEARTBURN

Roughly 60 million Americans experience heartburn every month.[474] Over the counter antacids are the drug of choice for these people, making antacids one of the most commonly used self-prescribed medications. The primary ingredients are calcium carbonate, magnesium, and aluminum salts in various combinations. The effect of antacids on the stomach is due to partial neutralization of gastric hydrochloric acid and inhibition of the enzyme pepsin.[475]

Using pharmacological acid suppression to heal peptic ulcers and to manage patients with GERD has been very successful, so much so that elective surgery for ulcer disease is now essentially non-existent.[476] But, the holistic question remains unanswered: Why is the need so great for antacids? What causes acid levels to rise?

All emotions have a direct relationship to a particular organ. Anxiety is the emotion most related to the stomach. Pressure situations, such as public speaking or doing anything new, can cause "butterflies in the stomach." Anxiety that is prolonged directly leads to disruption in stomach acid levels. Managing the everyday stresses of life, along with the free radicals bombardment of the civilized diet and environmental pollutants, is more than enough to cause changes in stomach acid levels.[477] In some people, stress has the opposite effect, causing a decrease in stomach acid levels. These people may in fact require hydrochloric acid (HCL) as a supplement. Many different nutrients, including fats, amino acids, and flavonoids, can have a healing effect on the lining of the stomach.[478]

PEPTIC ULCERS

A peptic ulcer is a sore in the lining of the stomach or duodenum. The duodenum is the first section of the small intestine. If peptic ulcers are found in the stomach, they're called gastric ulcers. If they're found in the duodenum, they're called duodenal ulcers. More than one ulcer is possible.

Approximately 25 million Americans suffer from peptic ulcer disease at some point in their lifetime. Each year, there are 500,000 to 850,000 new cases of peptic ulcer disease and more than one million ulcer-related hospitalizations.[479]

The pain of a peptic ulcer usually does the following:

- feels like a dull ache or burn.
- comes and goes for a few days or weeks.
- starts two to three hours after a meal.

- comes in the middle of the night when the stomach is empty.

- goes away after eating.

A specific bacteria, called helicobacter pylori (H. pylori), is responsible for two-thirds of all ulcers.[480][481] The other third is mostly from NSAIDS, like ibuprofen or acetaminophen. Most H. pylori infections are found in the duodenum.[482]

H. pylori is nothing to fool around with. It is associated with coronary artery disease and arteriosclerosis.[483] Long-term infection with H. pyloriis is directly linked to gastric cancer, the second most common cancer worldwide. In countries such as Colombia and China, H. pylori infects over half the population, beginning in childhood. In the United States, where H. pylori is less common in young people, gastric cancer rates have decreased since the 1930s.[484]

There is a double whammy with stomach acid and H. pylori. Ulcers are the result of too much acid, so using acid reducers is logical. But, here is the catch: lowering stomach acid makes the recurrence rate of an H. pylori infection much higher.[485] Therefore, balancing the PEP ST 1 with FBA, while at the same time eliminating any infection, is one's best option.

Antibiotics are the medical treatment of choice with an H. pylori infection. However, natural remedies are just as effective, and they are without the side effects that prolonged antibiotic use can bring. Flavonoids from plants,[486] the mineral bismuth citrate, and deglycyrrhizinated licorice root (DGL)[487] can all help heal ulcers and kill H. pylori.[488]

ACNE

Acne is a common skin condition of adolescence. For most, acne is temporary and without permanent damage. For around 42 million others, acne is moderate to severe, leaving both physical and emotional scars.

Acne is not just for teenagers. More than half of those with moderate to severe acne are women older than 25 years of age.[489]

The typical medical approach to acne includes oral contraceptives (OCs), antibiotics, and creams called retinoids.[490] If any of these are effective, then the source of the condition has just been revealed. OCs affect the hormones, antibiotics reduce infections and inflammation, and retinoids work directly on the clogged pores to reduce toxic build up. These are the same three key ingredients of functional illness (HIT) as discussed throughout *Hope for Health*. No matter the problem, HIT is usually involved.

The hormonal effect of oral contraceptives reduces acne lesions by increasing estrogen levels and by decreasing free testosterone levels. Blood sugar imbalances mainly fuel the inflammation of acne. Lastly, the toxins that damage skin come from both the outside, through what a person eats, drinks, and breathes, and through the inside, as a result of normal metabolic processes. What the liver cannot break down makes its way out through the largest organ of the body, the skin. It is the job of the liver to clean up hormones and to detoxify chemicals, making this organ a must-support in the treatment of acne. This topic is discussed in the chapter *Arthritic or Toxic?*

Stress is a major trigger of acne.[491] [492] The elements of civilized diet, an abundance of hormones, and learning how to grow up and become an adult form a perfect metabolic storm that ends up wreaking havoc on the skin of many individuals.

Rarely is diet ever discussed with acne. This is more than disappointing. The source of 95 percent of all chemical exposure, the reason for blood sugar imbalances and changes to the gut flora, and the instigator of most functional illness is not even considered. Medical doctors will point out that no foods have been proven to cause acne. This is only partially true. Foods do in fact cause acne, but not the same foods for the same people. Chocolate may promote acne by altering estrogen levels in one person, whereas tomatoes may lead to acne by increasing inflammation in another. Chances are, multiple simultaneous imbalances are present. FBA employs a holistic approach that systematically moves step by step from one PEP to the next, finding those in greatest need and fixing them with hormetic nutrients.

Acne means cleaning up the diet and changing behavior. It means getting well on the inside before skin improves on the outside. Since those seeking treatment for acne are mostly adolescents, asking them to make a 180-degree turn will pose a challenge. This is good. Challenges are opportunities to build self-confidence and to gain wisdom. Those young adults willing to embrace the changes necessary to get well on the inside will gain a sense of empowerment that moves them beyond their mere outward appearance and overflows into all aspects of health and life.

COLITIS OR CONSTIPATION? – LARGE INTESTINE 20

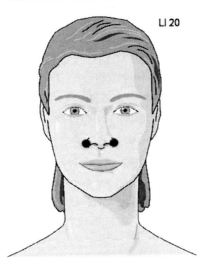

LI 20

Figure 39: Large Intestine 20

Related Neurotransmitter: GABA (low levels)

Organ or System: Large Intestine

Main Biomarkers: GABA, L-Glutamine, Glutamate

Common Hormetic Nutrients: Copper, B6, Magnesium, L-Tyrosine, Probiotics (bifidobacterium)

The PEP Large Intestine 20 is located at the lower sides of the nose in the crease where the nose transitions into the face. The neurotransmitter related to PEP LI 20 is gamma-aminobutyric acid, or GABA. When LI 20 causes a strong muscle to weaken, it means that GABA levels are too low. Looking at the figure below, GABA is synthesized from another neurotransmitter called glutamate.[493] Glutamate is excitatory and increases during times of stress. As the most ubiquitous inhibitory neurotransmitter in the brain, GABA acts like a brake, calming the chemicals of anxiety.

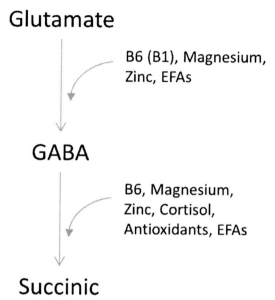

Figure 40: The GABA Pathway

Symptoms of low GABA include:

- Anxious or panic for no reason

- Excessive worry

- Feelings of being overwhelmed

- Feelings of dread or impending doom

- Guilt about everyday decisions

- Regular knots in the stomach

PROBIOTICS

Probiotics are the good bacteria that come from foods. They are part of the intestinal microflora, or flora for short. With around 100 trillion organisms and equaling about three to five pounds worth of material, the flora is like an organ unto itself. It is part of the body's natural defense,[494] and it acts as a barrier in the intestinal mucosa to prevent the attachment of pathogenic microorganisms. It is also part of the immune system.[495]

The benefits of probiotics are numerous. Allergies,[496] irritable bowel syndrome,[497] constipation, and diarrhea[498] are all alleviated when the right combination of probiotics are prescribed. Probiotics are also critical for the formation of vitamin B12 and biotin.[499]

One of the main reasons why people voluntarily take probiotics is because of constipation. In the United States, constipation is one of the most common gastrointestinal complaints. More than four million Americans have frequent constipation. The problem is much greater than this. Those reporting constipation most often are women and adults ages 65 and older.[500] However, many never seek help from their primary care physician, choosing instead to manage the constipation with over-the-counter laxatives.

Constipation occurs when the colon absorbs too little water or when the colon's muscle contractions are slow or sluggish, causing the stool to move through the colon too slowly. As a result, stools can become hard and dry. Finding out why there is dysfunction in the colon is determined through the PEPs with FBA. LI 20 is the PEP one would expect to find with constipation, but other PEPs may show up first. Once all are balanced, the constipation resolves. Why? Gut motility is related to many different systems. Stress (TW 23) and hormonal imbalances (CX 1) are two unrecognized causes of constipation. The common causes include the following things:

- Inadequate fiber in the diet
- Lack of physical activity (especially in the elderly)
- Medications

- Dairy products

- Irritable bowel syndrome

- Changes in life or routine, such as pregnancy, aging, and travel

- Abuse of laxatives

- Ignoring the urge to have a bowel movement

- Dehydration

- Problems with the colon and rectum

A multi-disciplinary approach, including nutrition, hydration, stress-management, and dietary considerations are often necessary to resolve the issue of constipation.[501] Probiotics can be helpful as well if the right ones are taken at the right time. Far too often people think just taking any probiotic will do. Most supplement store probiotics are a form called acidophilus. As their name suggests, these bacteria do well with acid. However, if the goal is to improve large intestine health, acidophilus will be of no help and may make matter worse.

The kind of probiotics that most benefit the large intestines are called bifidobacterium. These good bacteria do not like acid or oxygen. Ingesting them at a time when stomach acid levels are too high such as at breakfast, destroys many, since the highest amount of stomach acid is present between the hours of 7 a.m. to 11 a.m. Stomach acid is less at dinner and especially before bed. Therefore, once the right beneficial bacteria or combination is found through FBA, supplementation should be taken at least two hours after dinner.

PARASITES

A parasite is an organism that lives on or in a host. LI 20 could also indicate that a parasitic infection is active. Over 100 different types of parasitic worms can live in the human body. They range from microscopic in size to many feet long. Female worms can release 3,000 to 200,000 eggs per day depending on their type. Symptoms can range from uncomfortable to life threatening. Anemia, bloating, brain fog, fatigue, allergies, asthma, gas, digestive disorders, muscle and joint pain, nervousness, and skin rashes are commonly reported.

Parasites have been linked to almost every illness. Chronic parasitic infections drain the body of critical resources and destabilize the immune system. They can lead to secondary viral, bacterial, or fungal infections as well. Most people are living with parasites, unaware that the organisms are chipping away at their vitality. A healthy, strong immune system can and does eliminate most of these. However, if functional illness is already rampant, parasites may take up permanent residence.

Parasitic infections used to be thought of as the dread of the tropical regions. Actually, parasites live over much of the earth. Now, however, with worldwide travel commonplace, parasites are easily spread to different areas. Nationally reportable parasitic diseases include the following ones:

- Cryptosporidiosis,

- Cyclosporiasis,

- Giardiasis,

- Malaria, and

- Trichinellosis.

Treating Parasites

Some parasitic diseases are easily treated, and some are not. Generally, balancing vitamins and minerals simply will not do with a strong infection. A powerful herb like wormwood,[502] black walnut hull,[503] or Coptis Chinensis[504] is often required. Parasites often develop through various stages and life cycles, making them harder to kill. Whichever herbal remedy is found with FBA, it should be used for weeks after LI 20 no longer tests positive. This constant dose will insure that any developing parasites are eliminated as they mature.

HIGH SPIRITS OR HYPOXIA? – LUNG 1

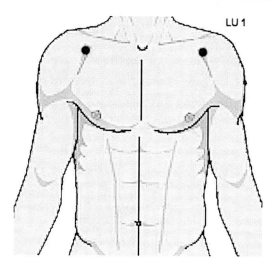

Figure 41: Lung 1

Related Neurotransmitter: GABA (high levels)

Organ or System: Respiratory System / Lungs

Main Biomarkers: GABA, L-Glutamine, Glutamate

Common Hormetic Nutrients: B6, Magnesium, Zinc

The PEP Lung 1 (LG 1) is located just to the inside of the shoulders and below the collarbone. PEP LG 1 is the point to look for if a patient has any respiratory problems, such as shallow breathing or asthma. Shallow breathing is often the result of anxiety and an overabundance of the chemicals of the fight-or-flight response. Together, these prevent the lungs from acquiring sufficient levels of oxygen and a state of hypoxia follows.

Respiration is possible because of the contraction of the diaphragm. If this specialized muscle fails to function properly, shallow breathing can ensue and so might another seemingly unrelated lung problem called a hiatal hernia. Chronic diaphragm stress can lead to overstretching of the opening around the esophagus, allowing the stomach to peer though. This is a painful problem that often mimics the symptoms of acid reflux. Simple in-office and at-home techniques to manually release the stomach can be very helpful for these patients.

ASTHMA

Asthma is a common chronic inflammatory disease of the airways. Symptoms include wheezing, coughing, chest tightness, and shortness of breath. Presently, 7.7 percent of Americans, or 17.5 million individuals, are diagnosed with Asthma.[505]

As one of the leading chronic childhood diseases in the United States, Asthma is a major cause of childhood disability. The prevalence of childhood asthma more than doubled from 1980 to the mid-1990s. It remains at historically high levels.[506] Like ADHD, which more than doubled in the same time period,[507] traditional medicine recognizes no known cause for either disease.

Testing with FBA has consistently shown that all patients with asthma need more cortisol, the natural anti-inflammatory steroid hormone from the adrenal glands. This finding is consistent with the primary treatment of MDs, who regularly prescribed synthetic steroids for asthma. These steroids include the medication prednisone and the inhaled steroids Qvar,™ Flovent,™ or Pulmicort.™ A steroid deficiency is not the primary cause of asthma, although in some it could be.

Cortisol is produced from the outer layers of the adrenal glands, known as the cortex. Children born with low-functioning or overworked adrenal glands will not produce sufficient levels of cortisol to manage lung inflammation. As mentioned several times previously, a current theory among alternative medicine doctors concerning the increasing levels of childhood illness is that immune-compromised and nutritionally deficient mothers are now giving birth to and raising immune-compromised and nutritionally deficient children. In 1960, only 1.8 percent of American children had a chronic health condition that limited their activities. In 2004, the rate rose to 7 percent.[508]

Concerning the PEP Lung 1, elevated GABA levels have a direct effect on the epithelial tissues of the lungs by increasing mucous production in asthma patients.[509] [510] This stimulatory effect is the opposite of the inhibitory effect of GABA in the brain and the central nervous system.[511] In the years to come, it will not be surprising to discover that many of the functions assigned to neurotransmitters are wrong or inadequate to explain all that they really do. The good news is everything need not be known about neurotransmitters in order to receive a maximum benefit from their activity, so long as they are properly made and metabolized. Overseeing these processes is a primary benefit of FBA.

Nutrition for Asthma and High GABA

Asthma is first and foremost a disease of inflammation. Controlling inflammation by balancing eicosanoid activity is therefore essential. This is done with precise essential fatty acids (EFAs) and other hormetic nutrients. Food allergies, chemical agents, artificial preservatives, and animal dander can all trigger an allergic reaction through the immune system. Refer to the chapter *The Foundation of Youth & Anti-Aging* for all the details.

In order to decrease total GABA levels, the prime movers B6, magnesium, and zinc are often required. Other natural substances also have a profound effect on asthma in general and GABA specifically. These include plant sterols, various antioxidants, and flavonoids.

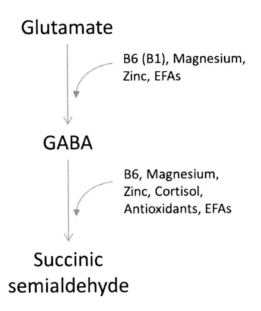

Figure 42: GABA Metabolism

Hidden Lung Issues

The body is a master compensator, finding ways to manage long-term issues. The longer it has managed a problem and not fixed it, the greater the probability it may not show up as expected through the PEPs. These are "hidden" issues. FBA practitioners are aware of this phenomenon and take steps to make the hidden problem manifest. Most of these issues are chronic drains on nutritional reserves, so getting rid of them is critical. In the lungs, they can often be brought out by placing a sample of GABA on or near the body.

There is another way to manifest lung issues with muscle testing. The patient touches PEP LG 1 with one hand, breaths in as deeply as possible, and holds his or her breath. A strong muscle is immediately tested. Then the patient exhales as much as possible and holds his or her breath out. If a strong muscle weakens after stressing the lungs this way, it reveals a hidden problem. Practitioners can often find chronic coughs from fungal, viral, or bacterial infections through this simple approach.

APPENDIX A - THE NEURO-EMOTIONAL COMPLEX

Hope for Health focuses primarily on inner body chemistry. However, false beliefs and trapped emotions acquired early in life or created over a lifetime greatly impact health. For many, physical illness first began as an emotional imbalance. If a patient's physical complaints fail to improve with FBA, it is likely the core problem has emotional roots that need tending. For the FBA practitioner, navigating the emotional labyrinth is not complex, but it can be all encompassing.

No event, past, present, or even thought about in the future, occurs without an emotional component. You are what you believe. In general, positive emotions promote healing and happiness, while negative emotions disrupt health in various ways by lowering the stress threshold. Both are contagious and have the potential to affect those people around an individual.

Psychoneuroimmunology is a field of study that recognizes the impact of emotions on physical health. Emotions such as grief, anxiety, anger, and pride direct human action more than people realize, often doing so on an unconscious level. This is the groundwork for future illness. Negative emotions can generate and fuel functional imbalances of every sort. A person must eliminate these negative emotions to restore health. When negative emotions cause functional imbalances, a neurological disturbance is present called a neuro-emotional complex (NEC). Traditional and complementary doctors will try in vain to resolve functional illness if NECs are present.

When an event or circumstance in the past or present is overwhelming or is "too much to deal with," an NEC can form. This is a coping mechanism that is protective for a time. However, an NEC can and will ultimately lead to functional imbalance. The origin of some NECs is obvious. The child who was molested, the teenager who didn't fit in, and the young adult who tried one experiment too many, all carry emotional bricks in life's backpack, loading them down and making every step harder than it should or needs to be.

An estimated 905,000 children were victims of child abuse or neglect in 2006.[512] Abused and neglected children are at least 25 percent more likely than those not abused or neglected to experience problems such as delinquency, teen pregnancy, low academic achievement, drug use, and mental health problems.[513]Abused and neglected children are 11 times more likely to be arrested for criminal behavior as juveniles, 2.7 times more likely to be arrested for violent and criminal behavior as adults, and 3.1 times more likely to be arrested for violent crimes.[514] Two-thirds of people in drug treatment programs reported being abused as children.[515]

Of course, a person does not need to have been abused or neglected in order to struggle with unconscious emotions. NECs can also develop from repeated minor events. From there, all it takes to turn a little problem into a big one is to do nothing. Leaving these negative emotions unaddressed means the little voice speaking healthy ideas—the one that is positive, productive, and contagious—is drowned out.

What once was an occasional reward, spawned by an "I deserve it because I worked so hard" attitude, soon became a habit, or more likely a coping mechanism. Giving in to the cravings of the body or to the desire for immediate gratification will not turn out well in the long run. Not just food and alcohol fit into this description. Entertainment; pleasures of all sorts; and, worst of all, bad beliefs and attitudes, all work together to sabotage a conscious wanting to manifest a healthy life. It is possible to smother health under excuses, justification, rationalization and full-fledged cognitive dissonance. This pattern fits all people in some way, meaning most have at least one NEC.

Negative emotions are not always bad, and positive emotions are not always good. A negative emotion, like inflammation in the body, sounds bad. However, positive and negative emotions both have important roles to play. Too much of either is crippling to the body. Positive emotions help people change direction and are highly motivating, often leading to great personal accomplishment. But, so are negative emotions. Some people see positive results from negative emotions. Being call "fat," "slow," "ugly," "dumb," or any other derogatory word may push one child toward self-pity and create a downward spiral of unproductive thoughts and unhealthy behaviors. In another child however, these same comments may be the catalyst to a life of effort, persistence, and healthy habits. Withstanding life's emotional body blows and fighting back with a flurry of counterpunches is a sign of good mental health.

Positive emotions alone can lead to imbalance, as well. The parent who showers with "love" but fails to restrain or correct his child immediately is likely to end up with a selfish little monster. Societies who fail to enforce boundaries and pass out entitlements by political reflex end up with selfish citizens (think student protests in France over a proposed increase in the retirement age from 60 to 62). These are both the result of too much positive emotion.

The law student who fails to pass his bar examination will be flooded with negative emotions: blame, anger, fear, etc. These are debilitating unless countered with even greater emotions like forgiveness, comfort, and love. There are three choices when it comes to negative emotions. The first two are healthy: correct the event that caused the emotion in the first place (pass the bar the next time) or replace the negative emotion with a positive one. Instead of beating himself up relentlessly for his own failures or blaming the test administrators, the time allotted, the location of the exam, and so on, the student could instead begin to strengthen himself emotionally for the next attempt by replacing negative emotions with positive ones. Instead of dwelling on negative thoughts, he could respond by telling himself, "I only missed by a few questions," "I know what to expect now," or "I am going to pass this time!" The third method for dealing with negative emotions, the one that leads to functional illness, is suppression—the main source of the NEC.

NEURO EMOTIONAL THERAPY – FIXING THE NEC

Once established, unconscious emotions are engrained. Like water coursing through a carved rock, negative emotional patterns have only one way to go when they pour forth. Making new routes by retraining the brain through thoughts, therapies, and actions allows positive emotions to take hold. These new routes allow the positive emotions to overcome the ones that promote an unhealthy physiology.

Recognizing a need beyond what psychology and psychiatry could provide, alternative health practitioners have developed many therapies to eliminate the NEC. Emotional Freedom Technique,[516] Neuro Emotional Therapy,[517] and Thought Field Therapy,[518] are examples. Each uses the idea that another, greater force can overcome a negative emotion. There are many important steps to undo the damage of NECs, not all of which are presented here. However, the details offered below are sufficient to gain an understanding of how the process works.

A person may have several NECs present at the same time. However, NECs, like everything else, follow a hierarchy. The emotion causing the greatest negative impact on health will show up first. In all likelihood, it will be the one associated with the first primary energetic point. Detecting the NEC is not difficult. If an NEC relates to anger, just saying the word "anger" aloud or having the patient think about the last time she was angry will make a strong muscle become weak.

Once a practitioner finds the NEC, he can begin treatment. While the patient maintains the thought of the emotional event, the practitioner will focus treatment toward all areas the emotion is affecting. Tapping the PEP or other acupressure points, adjusting spinal segments, and rubbing neurolymphatic organ reflexes, while maintaining the thought of the negative emotion, has an immediate dampening effect on the NEC. This is similar to the method used to desensitize allergies, as explained in the chapter *Allergies or Inflammation?* Dampening the NEC should take place in the office. The patient will need to work to retrain her brain. This means consciously overriding negative emotions throughout the day by using the most appropriate positive affirmation and by tapping the related PEP.

Treating the NEC

New beliefs are constructed and old beliefs deconstructed by thoughts and ideas. Before attempting to clear a patient from unconscious emotions, it is critical to know whether the individual is even ready to be set free. Many receive great benefit from being sick. Attention, assistance, and even money are available for those willing to manipulate others and ultimately themselves. There is little hope for balancing these folks. Those truly seeking help must first be clear of any emotional confusion, what is called, psychological reversal. This means that they will weaken to statements they shouldn't weaken to such as their name, or basic statements about themselves, or they may also weaken to healthy emotional statements such as:

- I am loveable.
- I am loving.
- I am loved.

When present, psychological reversal is an ongoing emotional self-sabotage. Straight-forward techniques are available to the FBA practitioner, which undo reversals and confusion so that emotional healing can progress.

The PEPs and Their Emotions

As shown in the table on the opposite page, all primary energetic points have a direct connection with a specific neurotransmitter, as well as having a direct association with an emotion. This knowledge is very helpful when it comes to correcting the NEC.

Whichever PEP is found, its related emotion can be evaluated to see if an NEC is present. For example, if the PEP large intestine 21 causes a strong muscle to weaken, the patient should say the words, "despair," "apathy," and "hopeless." If a strong muscle becomes weak again to any of these words, then an NEC is present. One way to eliminate the NEC is to tap the PEP for one or more minutes while stating the counteractive affirmation. For instance, to counteract the negative emotion "hopeless," a patient could state, "I am hopeful in my life (my career, with my relationships, etc. "Likewise, if someone has a fear of failure, a positive affirmation for her may be saying, "I will overcome (accomplish) all obstacles that prevent health and happiness. "

PEP	Emotion	Neurotransmitter
Spleen 21	Agitation / Overwhelmed	↑ Histamine
Stomach 1	Listless / Lethargic	↓ Histamine
Circulation/Sex 1	Manic / Bewilderment	↑ Aspartate/Glutamate
Triple Warmer 23	Panic / Trapped	↓ Aspartate/Glutamate
Liver 14	Pride / Scorn	↑ Acetyl Choline
Gall Bladder 1	Guilt / Blame / Judgmentalness	↓ Acetyl Choline
Governing Vessel 27	Lust / Desire	↑Dopamine
Conception Vessel 24	Grief / Regret	↓ Dopamine
Heart 1	Tension / Irritation	↑ Norepinephrine
Small Intestine 19	Indecisive / Laziness	↓ Norepinephrine
Kidney 27	Anxiety / Fear	↑ Serotonin
Bladder 1	Shame / Humiliation	↓ Serotonin
Lung 1	Anger / Hate	↑ GABA
Large Intestine 20	Apathy / Despair	↓ GABA

Whatever the affirmation, it needs to prevent the PEP and the negative emotions from causing a strong muscle to weaken. If it does, the patient should say this affirmation several times per day but not sheepishly. Repetition and intensity will make a home for the new idea in the brain through a process called neuroplasticity. Eventually, these new healthy thoughts will turn into new healthy actions.

APPENDIX B - EXERCISE

In the same way that love covers over the wrongs done to people by others, exercise covers a multitude of dietary and lifestyle transgressions. No single therapy has as great an impact on the body as exercise. The respiratory, immune, lymphatic, digestive, musculoskeletal, energy, emotional, and every other system all benefit from proper, regular exercise.[519]

Everyone knows about exercise for strengthening the heart and lungs and for building muscle. But, there is so much more to it. New research has demonstrated that muscle contraction through sustained exercise increases the level of immune chemicals, called myokines, which help fight off infections and speed up metabolism.[520] This phenomenon is so prevalent that many are now considering muscles as an extension of the immune system.[521] [522] Likewise, proper exercise helps burn fat, which releases appetite-suppressing and satiety chemicals, called lipokines.[523]

Doing Too Much

There is such a thing as detrimental exercise. It is generally the "no pain, no gain" approach that poses the greatest threat. This is the type of exercise you can expect to find when working with a personal trainer or after signing up to lose weight on reality television. Strenuous exercise under prolonged emotional stress can promote steady weight gain in the form of fat.[524] Strenuous exercise often overworks the heart[525] and leads to an increased risk of sudden cardiac arrest.[526] It can also lead to tissue damage in the joints and a worsening of the already health-snatching fight-or-flight response.[527]

The "no-pain, no-gain" approach can work for some, but for most it is damaging or simply will not last. Remember, a personal trainer is probably not a dropout from the mechanical engineering department at MIT. More likely, he is a former athlete of some renown, blessed with an abundance of fast twitch muscle fibers (think NFL linebacker). When he does a strenuous workout, his body responds (at least until around age 45).

Logically, although inaccurately, he takes the same set of routines that work for him and translates them to his clients. Only about one third of new exercisers will have a positive response to strenuous exercise alone. The general rule is *a person who is healthy may use all forms of exercise, but not all exercise makes a person healthy.*

All people can respond to strenuous exercise, but first things first. Everyone must build up the aerobic metabolism to make sure fat burning is the primary means of making fuel before proceeding on to other, more intense forms of exercise. People will get no argument from most when they are told that they need to make fat burning their primary goal. That is why they joined the gym in the first place.

Amazingly, 6 of the top 10 causes of death directly relate to being overweight or obese. This means that almost 71 percent of all deaths in the U.S. each year are related to a preventable problem that costs around $150 billion annually.[528] Using fat as the body's primary fuel is the healthiest metabolism possible. The number one way to shut off this source of unlimited energy is with a blood sugar problem, such as insulin resistance — a problem created by the dietary habits of industrialized people.

Yesterday's dietary rules stated that good nutrition was merely the right ratio of fats, carbohydrates, and proteins; that a multivitamin or B-complex was all the supplemental nutrition one might need, if any at all; and that losing weight was simply a matter of calories-in vs. calories-out.[529] Yesterday is gone. Doctors who practice functional medicine regularly accept new patients, whose primary complaint is that they eat very little, exercise a great deal, and yet are exhausted and cannot lose weight. Some are in fact gaining weight. With each pass of the mirror, these patients observe an expanding body of evidence that conflicts with commonly held nutritional theories and thus realize that something important is missing from the calorie/exercise equation.

FITNESS VS. HEALTH

A fit person is not necessarily healthy, nor is the healthy person necessarily fit. When an athlete allows his body to adapt to the various stressors he has placed upon it, the body can most certainly become fit. The fit athlete, having trained his body appropriately, is able to perform strenuous and astounding feats, yet this benefit will most likely come at the expense of other tissues and often at the expense of health itself.

On a personal note, before I ever knew anything about exercise, nutrition, and the adverse effects of stress, I was able to maintain a high degree of fitness from regular exercise. Basketball and weight lifting were an integral part of my week. If a stranger looked at me, he would think I was in good shape and healthy. Yet, with any sort of sustained stress, I would usually get sick. Other signs were also present, including chronic mucus in my throat, frequent sniffling, sneezing, achy joints from time to time, swelling in my left knee, and allergies to cats, dogs, and various foods (all of this before I was 33!). Although I was able to lift weights for two hours at a time and play basketball half of the day, I was still plagued with numerous symptoms. I may have been fit, but I was not healthy.

In my opinion, most exercise programs that utilize the "no pain, no gain" approach exclusively are unintentionally producing the same problems among the public. It is not uncommon to hear of a well-known athlete having his career cut short due to nagging injuries or even by unexpected death while training. People can assume certain deficiencies of hormetic nutrients will arise when training for fitness and not for health. These deficiencies will eventually result in significant physiologic imbalance. This is because fitness training places heavy burdens on the body's anaerobic (sugar burning) system while neglecting the more important aerobic (oxygen and fat burning) system.

THE ANAEROBIC SYSTEM

The anaerobic system is vital to life. It provides quick energy by using stored blood sugar (glycogen) for fuel. No oxygen is required with the anaerobic system. Many organs benefit from immediate access to glucose, but none more so than the brain, which requires a steady diet of glucose in order to operate. Very small amounts of glycogen are available for use by the muscles at any given time. That is why weight training "sets" last only a short period before the muscles "burn out." Too much anaerobic training can cause chemical imbalances that lead to injury and eventually illness. Weight training, sprinting, fast jogging, and most other sports are forms of anaerobic exercise.

Two types of muscle fibers, named "fast" and "slow," make up the body. Fast fibers are also called anaerobic fibers, while slow fibers are called aerobic fibers. Genetics often determine how much of each are present. Through training, an athlete can change the function of a particular fiber, making a slow fiber act like a fast fiber and vice versa. Once training has stopped, however, the cells gradually return to their previous genetically determined state.

Sprinters and bodybuilders do not have the same number of slow fibers as long distance athletes. Instead, they have more fast fibers. All athletes, which includes everyone who exercises regularly, have certain special needs. However, it is interesting to note that athletes participating in fast fiber sports perform better if they train their slow fibers, as well, according to the method described below.

THE AEROBIC SYSTEM

Aerobic training (light jogging, easy swimming, easy biking etc.) is extremely beneficial in the promotion of health. In order to engage the aerobic system, exercise must take place within a certain, low heart rate range. The aerobic system relies on great amounts of oxygen in order to produce energy, and the major fuel used when training aerobically is fat. The same amount of fat contains more than twice as much potential fuel as do carbohydrates (sugars). Therefore, when engaging the aerobic system during exercise, energy accumulation becomes more efficient as fat is burned. Not only should fat be the fuel of choice for energy, it is also the one most people want to get rid of in the first place. Too much aerobic training is possible, but rare. For the most part, aerobic activity fulfills all the promises of exercise, while additionally promoting fat loss and increasing energy.

TARGET HEART RATE

The body switches from fat burning to sugar burning at a specific heart rate. Therefore, the purchase of a heart rate monitor is highly recommended. Once the heart rate exceeds a certain range, the aerobic system is disengaged and the anaerobic system takes over. This means stored sugars, not stored fat will become the fuel of choice. All aerobic benefit is potentially lost when training at a non-aerobic heart rate (too fast).

A heart rate monitor will beep when the individual exceeds the fat-burning range. Heart rate monitors are very simple to use and usually include two pieces: a wrist piece that tells the rate of beats per minute (doubles as a watch when not in use) and a strap that goes around the chest which picks up the electrical signals given off by the heart with each beat. Most sports stores sell heart rate monitors for less than $100.00.

Finding Your Target Heart Rate Range:
The following information is adapted from the book *In Fitness and In Health*, authored by Dr. Phil Maffetone, a well-known Applied Kinesiologist who has successfully worked with thousands of patients and many elite athletes to improve their aerobic capacity and overall performance. (www.philmaffetone.com)

Subtract your age from the number **180**.

Then add or subtract from this number based upon the following:

- Recovering from a major illness, surgery, or taking daily medication.....**subtract 10**
- Have not exercised before; have exercised but have been injured or are regressing; experience frequent colds or flu, or are under high stress.....**subtract 5**
- Exercising for up to two years without any real problems and have not had colds or flu more than once or twice per year...**subtract 0**
- Exercising for more than two years without any real problems and have been making progress in your program or competition.....**add 5**

This final number is the upper end of your heart rate range. To find the lower end, subtract 10 points from the upper number.

For example, a person would calculate the heart rate number for a 50-year-old-man to be 130 (180-50). But, he also rarely exercises and gets the flu and/or a cold most years, so the person would need to subtract another 5 points to end up with an upper number of 125. The overall range is 10 points below the upper number or 115-125 bpm. This is his fat-burning heart rate zone. An individual can set any heart rate monitor for this range. When exercising pushes the heart above this range, a beep will sound. Exercising exclusively within this ten point range will yield the greatest aerobic return and generate the highest level of fat-burning.

What to Expect

When first using a heart rate monitor, most people, including regular runners and those who exercise two or three times per week with no apparent difficulty, are shocked by how quickly their heart rate exceeds its maximum range. Not surprisingly, these same patients showed many signs of adrenal gland fatigue and nagging injuries. They needed to slow down in order to build a solid aerobic base first. The good news is after training in their aerobic range for only a short period of time, they were able to resume their previous running course and speed but with a much slower (healthier) heart rate.

Selecting a Program

An aerobic program should be performed at least three times per week for 30 minutes each session. As the training progresses, the person can increase the frequency (to five, sometimes six, times per week) and time (to 60 minutes or more).

Walking is the best way to start and will be the only choice for most people. Those currently doing some form of exercise may be able to lightly jog or swim. Whatever the exercise, it should involve the large muscles of the legs, be continuous for the determined amount of time, and always stay in or below the target heart rate range.

The ultimate goal with training in the heart rate zone is to improve aerobic function, which means using oxygen to burn fat. A light sweat, easy breathing, and a feeling of not having done too much once exercise is finished are all good signs that training was below the maximum heart rate. Another sign is the presence of sore muscles. Since most people have inadvertently exercised too hard, they have over trained their fast fibers and neglected their slow fibers. Training at a lower heart rate uses the slow (fat burning) fibers almost exclusively. Using previously unused muscles makes them temporarily sore. This is good and will soon pass.

The Emotional Component

Wanting to exercise can be just as important as doing it. An individual should always address the emotional component in any activity. Therefore, pick a route that is enjoyable, a time of day that is convenient, clothing that is comfortable, and an attitude that is appreciative and determined. Tying productive emotions into any new routine or discipline helps to get through the tougher stages and encourages progress.

Warm Up, Cool Down, and Stretching

Warming up and stretching are essential, but they are not the same thing. Warming up should always happen first and is as simple as a slow easy walk for 10 minutes. It is necessary in order to prepare the body for exercise and to prevent injury. Warming up also begins the fat-burning process by promoting the release of free-floating fatty acids, the desired energy source.

Up to 80 percent of the blood in the organs will be transferred to the muscles during exercise. Warming up prior to intense exercise allows this fluid transfer to happen gradually. This is important for another reason. Exercise generates vast quantities of metabolic waste products. Warming up ensures that a sufficient amount of blood is circulating prior to exercise, so these by-products can be shuttled to the liver for detoxification and elimination.

After the brief warm-up period, stretching may be performed. The added circulation from the warm-up period allows for greater elasticity and flexibility of the tissues during a stretch, decreasing the chance for injury. A person should not stretch through the point of pain and should not bounce when stretching. Stretching beyond the normal range of motion may temporarily increase flexibility, but it also leads to micro injury.

The best form of stretching is a static-active stretch. This means moving slowly to a point of resistance, and contracting the opposite muscle for 10 - 20 seconds. For example, to stretch the muscles on the back of the right leg (hamstrings), an individual would mildly contract the muscles on the front of the right leg (quads) for about 20 seconds. Contracting one group of muscles has the neurologic effect of turning off or relaxing its opposing group.

The cool down is just as important as the warm up. Cooling down allows a gentle return of the blood to the various organs. Stopping suddenly after exercise causes the blood to rush quickly into the organs, bringing with it an abundance of exercise-induced waste products. Since most blood is stored within the organs during times of inactivity, without a cool down, chemical waste products may amass. The potential toxic buildup, if severe enough, could mean a large portion of the aerobic benefits from the exercise are lost. At the end of the walk/jog, simply reduce the exercise pace gradually until the heart rate is about 10 - 20 beats above the resting heart rate. This process is all that is needed and should only take about 10 minutes.

MAXIMUM AEROBIC FUNCTION TEST (MAF)

It is always a good idea to monitor exercise progress. After a few weeks of heart rate training, positive signs will be present, such as feeling better, not being as tired, having more energy, gaining resistance to sickness, improved sleep patterns, etc. These subjective findings are important, but a maximum aerobic function test (MAF) to check for objective changes is critical, as well.

A person should choose a distance, such as 8 or 10 times around the local high school track, and jog or walk the entire distance while within their target heart rate range, speeding up or slow down as necessary. Once the distance is completed, she should record the time. After two or three weeks, she should repeat the MAF test. Be sure that the conditions are similar for each test. The results from a calm still day may be different than those from a wet and windy day. If, after the next MAF test, the individual can cover the same distance in less time while staying within the target heart rate range, then the aerobic system is improving.

The opposite can be done, as well. Choose a specific amount of time to perform an exercise and measure the total distance. Progress means being able to go further on a subsequent test within the same amount of time. These tests are important emotionally because they quantitatively demonstrate progress, which encourages continued exercise. People should perform a MAF test every three or four weeks.

Most will find that they improve rather quickly, and that they need to progress from walking to a slow jog in order to not fall below their heart rate range. If improvement has not occurred, other variables should be considered. Are sickness, additional stress, inadequate rest, or too many bad foods, contributing to poor progress? If so, these must be addressed. It may also be a wise idea to seek help from an FBA practitioner at this time. It may be as simple as a few minor tweaks to get health back on track.

Summary

- Train aerobically for three months without anaerobic exercise.
- Do not exceed your maximum heart rate at any time during your workout.
- When training without a heart rate monitor, an individual should only exercise at a pace where he notices little exertion.
- Warm up.
- Stretch.
- Cool down.
- Do monthly MAF tests to ensure progress.

APPENDIX C - ENERGY TO BURN?

The complaint of fatigue is one of the top three reasons why people visit their doctors. However, this one symptom, is proof in itself that the medical model of treating parts is flawed. When the thyroid medicine fails, to which specialist does the MD refer his patients for fatigue? The vitalogist? The oomphologist? Every time an MD hears the complaint of fatigue, it is a direct reminder that the traditional form of health care, the one they have practiced for decades and spent hundreds of thousands of dollars to master and propagate, is insufficient. Fatigue, and nearly every other aliment, is multi-faceted – enlisting numerous systems all at the same time.

From a functional medicine perspective, a person who thinks his energy is "fine" is probably not operating in his highest gear. The body only needs about 10 to 20 percent of its total energy to navigate civilized life, including waking up, washing, working at a desk, watching TV, etc. Neurological function, digestion, repair, detoxification, metabolism, immune system function and other internal occupations carried on automatically via the autonomic nervous system use the majority of the energy required on a daily basis. It is in these areas that things break down first.

The creation of energy is dependent upon numerous mechanisms and cellular interactions that must operate simultaneously in order to achieve one ultimate goal: the generation of an essential molecule called ATP. The entire energy-making system is a metabolic maze that is vulnerable on many fronts. As has been described throughout *Hope for Health*, the primary assault comes through poor digestion, immune system disruptions, blood sugar mismanagement and hormone imbalances – all leading to cellular inflammation. With FBA, a practitioner can track the entire energy pathway, which contains four steps within two phases, from start to finish.

WHAT IS ENERGY?

Without food (macro-nutrition) we would die of starvation after 40 days. Without water, we could last perhaps a week. Without oxygen life would cease in just minutes. If all the ATP were suddenly removed from the body, survival would last no more than three seconds.

ATP is one molecule of adenosine with three phosphate groups attached to it. All reactions, including intracellular, extracellular or otherwise, are dependent upon the donation of a single phosphate group from the ATP molecule. ATP forms by adding a phosphate molecule to adenosine to make the single (mono) phosphate molecule AMP. Adding another phosphate makes the two (di) phosphate ADP. The addition of a third phosphate completes the process to form ATP. Energy production in the form of ATP happens trillions of times per second. ATP can give or take phosphate molecules. Giving away phosphate molecules is the easy part. Gathering them back again is where the trouble lies. If there is an abundance of ATP, then there is energy to burn. However, the road to energy has many speed bumps.

Energy production takes place in two phases, each with two steps. The goal of the first phase, called glycolysis, is to take the food a person eats and turn it into blood sugar (glucose). Then the body converts glucose into a molecule called acetyl CoA. The second phase takes the newly-made acetyl CoA and makes a bundle of ATP with the help of oxygen. This is called oxidative phosphorylation. If all goes well, one glucose molecule can move through both phases and create a total of 38 energy-making ATP molecules.

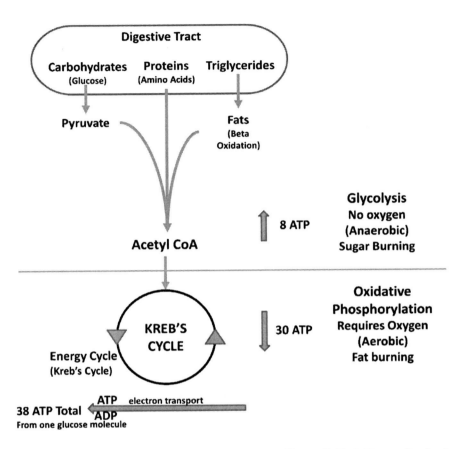

Figure 43: Basic Energy Production

The figure above illustrates the basic steps of the energy cycle beginning with Step 1: the digestion of proteins, carbohydrates and fats. The body must break down each of these macromolecules in order to make the end product, acetyl CoA. Getting from one glucose molecule to acetyl CoA creates only 8 of the desired 38 ATP molecules. Once acetyl CoA is made, the body must transport it into the Kreb's cycle. This is Step 2. In Step 3, acetyl CoA spins inside the Kreb's cycle. The round-about process transforms acetyl CoA into a series of eight different molecules. The eighth is soon reformed back into the first, beginning the cycle again. This may sound futile, but it is not. The process creates another two ATP molecules, as well as a host of very important chemicals used throughout the body and the brain. With two-thirds of energy production completed, the body has generated a total of 10 of the desired 38 ATP molecules. Step 4, the final step, produces the lion's share of ATP. In this step, called the electron transport chain, the phosphate molecules are added to the stockpile of ADP, generating the final 28 ATP molecules.

Energy Zapped

Each step of the energy pathway has specific requirements. If these requirements are not met, then energy production can go no further. If the digestive system is compromised, proteins, carbohydrates and fats are not properly broken down in Step 1, resulting in low levels of acetyl CoA. This is like a new car; the parts are all put together, but without some gas in the tank, it won't be going anywhere. So, what if digestion is working fine and there is gas in the tank? The next potential problem is a hormonal one. Step 2 is dependent upon proper functioning of the thyroid gland. If the thyroid gland is under-functioning, then the body will not shuttle acetyl CoA into the Kreb's cycle. This is why people with hypothyroidism complain of being tired. The analogy at this step would be a broken fuel pump—the gas is in the tank, but the fuel cannot be pushed into the pistons.

In order to spin the Kreb's cycle, many important ingredients must be present. Step 3 requires specific B vitamins and the right form of magnesium. These are the sparks of the energy cycle. Fuel in the pistons without a spark from the plugs is useless. Finally, Step 4. The engine in a car provides the power, and the transmission makes the axel spin and the wheels turn. If Steps 1 to 3 are working, then the body is moving down the road. If the transmission slips, Step 4 will never get into high gear. This step requires the emperor of all nutrients: oxygen. The red blood cells, with the help of iron or vitamin B12, carry oxygen. When a person's oxygen supply is low, she will always feel tired. This is the case with any form of anemia.

All of the above may have sounded complicated, but here is the good news: A handful of hormetic nutrients are sufficient to handle all the steps in both phases and to make the energy system function properly.

The FBA practitioner can, in a matter of minutes, evaluate each of the steps and the nutrients they require.

BURN FAT, NOT MUSCLE

If the body, for whatever reason, fails to move from Phase I (glycolysis) into Phase II (oxidative phosphorylation), then the total energy supply will be around 20 percent of its designed capacity. This degree of energy deficit requires emergency measures, and the body is forced to take them. In an attempt to generate at least some of the necessary ATP to stay alive, the body resorts to a process called gluconeogenesis—the creation of glucose from other molecules. The radical but common method is through the destruction of muscle tissue in order to yield lactic acid and amino acids. In other words, the body "eats" its own muscle. The amino acids from this process can then enter into the Kreb's cycle. Through a series of steps, the body can then use lactic acid to make glucose. Obviously, this method of energy creation is less than desirable. It is however, the regular metabolic state for people who over-train, are under excessive stress, or have blood sugar imbalances.

The inflammation from overtraining or free radical damage produces an abundance of immune chemicals called cytokines. These further disrupt Phase II metabolism and prevent weight loss because they prevent the fat-burning chemical, hormone sensitive lipase, from doing its job.

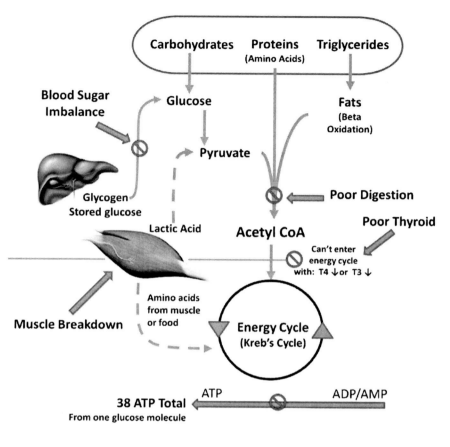

Figure 44: Potholes in the Pathway

The example is all too common. The once-fit female in her twenties and thirties turns forty, and everything seems to fall apart. The signs of the shift were there all along. In some cases, the competitive spirit and the no pain, no gain approach allowed a person to ignore the signs. The athlete presses through her workouts, expecting that the same results of a tight tummy and better fitting clothes are just a few less bites and a few extra reps away. But things are not as they once were.

A lifetime of forcing the body to respond and adapt to exercise and/or emotional stress has led to the poor regulation of critical energy systems and to the depletion of nutrients, which are essential for fat conversion, stored sugar utilization, brain neurotransmitter balance, insulin regulation and immune system equilibrium. Now, as she once again calls upon her metabolism to switch into a higher gear, her body is unable to respond.

Gradually, despite extensive effort on her part, the fat increases and the muscle decreases. Like quicksand, the more she struggles to free herself through the tried-and-true methods, the more she can't. She is stuck in Phase I. Sadly, this is not the end of the bad news. The same stressors that poisoned Phase I have likely contaminated Phase II, as well. This means that she cannot turn ADP into ATP–the highest ATP-yielding part of the entire cycle.

Remember, if energy production becomes stuck anywhere before the final step from ADP to ATP, the net loss in total energy can be as much as 80 percent. Clearly, an energy level this meager equates to a poor quality of life. To avoid this dismal state, the body would surely avail itself of any complementary measures should they be obtainable. They are, and it does. But the cost is high.

Escaping Glycolysis – Phase I Repair

Over-eating and being over-stressed and over-tired are the reasons most people are stuck in glycolysis–storing fat and burning muscle. To escape Phase I and move into the Kreb's cycle, a practitioner must answer five questions.

- *Is the body properly mobilizing fat?* Lipolysis is the process of releasing fat from its storage site, the adipose tissue. The process requires many nutrients for this to happen, and too much adrenaline, a powerful stress hormone, can hinder the process. The likely hormetic nutrients that aid in this step are carnitine, magnesium phosphate, niacin (B3) in one of its many forms, and the enzyme lipase.

- *Is the body correctly utilizing fat?* Once the tissue releases fat, it circulates in the blood stream as triglycerides. The body breaks triglycerides into their smaller parts to eventually wind up as acetyl CoA. If the practitioner finds a deficiency here, a person may need a specific form of vitamin B3 (niacin). Niacin has several activated forms. Patients need one called NADH about 70 percent of the time and NADP and NADPH the other 30 percent.

- *Is the thyroid happy?* The two major thyroid hormones (T3 and T4) help with the movement of acetyl CoA into the Kreb's cycle. It is rare to find a thyroid problem in isolation. Often, the thyroid is secondarily troubled by too much insulin, which interferes with the hookup locations of T3 and T4, called receptor sites. If T3 is the primary hormonal issue, then selenium is often an important nutrient. If T4 is the problem, then iodine is critical (except in the cases of auto-immune thyroid, called Hashimoto's disease).

- *Is the body properly making glycogen?* After meals, left-over glucose is likely. This extra glucose is either stored in the liver, muscles and kidneys as a substance called glycogen, or the body converts it into fat. Some, because of too much adrenaline, do not store glycogen properly, making blood sugar reserves too low. This becomes apparent between meals when the body is looking for its primary fuel, glucose, in order to feed the brain and other tissues. If there are insignificant amounts of glycogen, then hypoglycemic symptoms, such as shaking, lightheadedness, or strong sweet cravings, are likely. The antidote to this problem is often to increase cortisol levels by repairing tired adrenal glands and by finding the appropriate form of calcium or vitamin B1 or B12, as well as certain trace minerals.

- *Is the body correctly utilizing glycogen?* There may be plenty of glycogen in the storage compartments of the liver, muscles, and kidneys, but if the cabinets are locked, it is of no value. Vitamin B6, in its activated form, pyridoxal-5-phosphate, is the key. The body will also require adrenaline for glycogen release. However, due to multiple forms of stress, most people are already full of this excitatory substance.

Finishing Strong – Phase II Repair

Phase II is made up of the Kreb's cycle and the electron transport chain. Here are the two most likely scenarios for a breakdown in one or both of these steps:

- *Does the person have enough B vitamins?* The Kreb's cycle is the least affected of the four steps of the energy pathway for a variety of reasons. The ones who need it supported the most are the athletes/weekend warriors. Most people—the ones who think they need it the most—are too sick to handle a B complex or even a multi-vitamin. The temporary energy boost felt from these supplements is more like a caffeine-buzz than a healthy lift to the energy system, and they can produce unwanted side effects. However, for the athlete, the demand for proper levels of B vitamins is high, and without them, the Kreb's cycle suffers.

- *Is the body adding the final phosphate?* As shown above, ADP must, with the addition of a third phosphate, be made into ATP. Here too, insulin is the primary disruptor. In this stage, however, iron and vitamin B12 become critical. Without iron and B12, the body does not properly carry oxygen throughout the cell and the mitochondria where the energy creation takes place. To correct the problem, the patient usually needs one of the activated forms of B12, called adenosylcobalamin, and the mineral, iron phosphate. The last nutrient of importance for energy production is magnesium. Remember, there are over 2,500 known enzymes in the human body and 70 percent of these require magnesium. Of course, not just any magnesium will do. In the case of low energy, magnesium phosphate is often the best choice.

Finding the hormetic nutrients necessary to dissect the energy pathway and restart the metabolic engine is not difficult. Energy restoration becomes complicated when trying to find what caused the nutrient deficiencies in the first place. To do so, a practitioner needs to evaluate individual systems through the primary reflex points. As is true with any part of health restoration, repairs can quickly become undone if a person fails to make certain lifestyle changes. The incorporation of a hypoglycemic diet and the initiation of an aerobic-only exercise program are both critical for energy-cycle correction.

BIBLIOGRAPHY

[1] National Health Interview Survey, 1997-March 2010.
http://www.cdc.gov/nchs/data/nhis/earlyrelease/201009_11.pdf

[2] Most People Think They Are Healthy.
http://www.netdoctor.co.uk/interactive/news/theme_news_detail.php?id=190913
28&tab_id=103

[3] National Health Interview Survey, 1997-March 2010.
http://www.cdc.gov/nchs/data/nhis/earlyrelease/201009_11.pdf

[4] Deaths and Mortality. http://www.cdc.gov/nchs/fastats/deaths.htm

[5] Mental Disorders Affect 1 in 4 People. The World Health Report 2001.
http://www.who.int/inf-pr-2001/en/pr2001-42.html

[6] Life Expectancy. Center for Disease Control.
http://www.cdc.gov/nchs/fastats/lifexpec.htm

[7] Cohen, S., Tyrrell, D. A., and Smith, A. P. (1991). Psychological Stress and Susceptibility to the Common Cold. The New England Journal of Medicine 325(9), 606-12.

[8] Chrousos, G. P. and Gold, P. W. (1992).The Concepts of Stress and Stress System Disorders. Overview of Physical and Behavioral Homeostasis. JAMA 267(Mar 4), 1244-52.

[9] Gur A, Oktayoglu P. Central Nervous System Abnormalities in Fibromyalgia and Chronic Fatigue
Syndrome: New Concepts in Treatment. Curr Pharm Des. 2008;14(13):1274-94.

[10] Buskila D, Press J. Neuroendocrine Mechanisms in Fibromyalgia-Chronic Fatigue. Best Pract Res ClinRheumatol. 2001 Dec;15(5):747-58.

[11] Fibromyalgia: Poorly Understood; Treatments are Disappointing. Prescrire Int. 2009 Aug;18(102):169-73.

[12] Crofford LJ. The hypothalamic-Pituitary-Adrenal Stress Axis in Fibromyalgia and Chronic
Fatigue Syndrome. Z Rheumatol. 1998;57Suppl 2:67-71.

[13] Fossel M. Cell Senescence in Human Aging and Disease. *Ann N Y Acad Sci*. 2002 Apr;959:14-23.

[14] Hayflick L. (1965). The Limited in Vitro Lifetime of Human Diploid Cell Strains. Exp. Cell Res. 37 (3): 614-636.

[15] Oz, Mehmet, Roizen, M. You: The Owner's Manual: An Insider's Guide to The Body That Will Make You Healthier and Younger. Harper Collins Publishers; 2005.

[16] Benn, P. A. Specific Chromosome Aberrations in Senescent Fibroblast Cell Lines Derived from Human Embryos. Am J Hum Genet 28(5): 465-473 (1976);

[17] Boukamp, P., S. Popp, et al. (2005). Telomere-dependent Chromosomal Instability. J Investig Dermatol Symp Proc 10(2): 89-94 (2005).

[18] Meza-Zepeda, L. A., A. Noer, et al. High-resolution Analysis of Genetic Stability of Human Adipose Tissue Stem Cells Cultured to Senescence. J Cell Mol Med 12(2): 553-263 (2008)

[19] Andrews, Bill. Curing Aging. http://www.sierrasciences.com/telomere/index.html

[20] Funk, et al. Telomerase Expression Restores Dermal Integrity to in Vitro-Aged Fibroblasts in a Reconstituted Skin Model. Experimental Cell Research, 2000

[21] Bodnar, et al. Extension of Life-Span by Introduction of Telomerase into Normal Human Cells. Science, 1998.

[22] Choi J, Fauce SR, Eff ros RB. Reduced Telomerase Activity in Human T lymphocytes Exposed to Cortisol. Brain Behav Immun. 2008;22: 600–05.

[23] Richter T, Zglinicki T. A Continuous Correlation between Oxidative Stress and Telomere Shortening in Fibroblasts. Exp Gerontol. 2007;42: 1039–42

[24] Epel ES, Blackburn EH, Lin J, et al. Accelerated Telomere Shortening in Response to Life Stress. *Proc Natl Acad Sci USA*. 2004;101: 17312–15.

[25] Jennings B, Ozanne S, Hales CN. Nutrition, Oxidative Damage, Telomere Shortening, and Cellular Senescence: Individual or Connected Agents of Aging?. *Mol Gen & Metab*. 2000; 71:32-42

[26] Passos JF, von Zglinicki T. Mitochondria, Telomeres and Cell Senescence. *Exp Gerontol*. 2005 Jun;40(6):466-72.

[27] Passos JF, Saretzki G, von Zglinicki T. DNA Damage in Telomeres and Mitochondria during Cellular Senescence: Is There a Connection? *Nucleic Acids Res*. 2007;35(22):7505-13

[28] Liu L, Trimarchi JR, Smith PJ, et al. Mitochondrial Dysfunction Leads to Telomere Attrition and Genomic Instability. *Aging Cell*. 1 (2002), pp. 40–46.

[29] Tentolouris N, Nzietchueng R, Cattan V, et al. White Blood Cells Telomere Length is Shorter in Males with Type 2 Diabetes and Microalbuminuria. *Diabetes Care*. 2007 Nov;30(11):2909-15.

[30] Adaikalakoteswari A, Balasubramanyam M, Ravikumar R, et al. Association of Telomere Shortening with Impaired Glucose Tolerance and Diabetic Macroangiopathy. *Atherosclerosis*. 2007 Nov;195(1):83-9.

[31] Cherkas LF, Hunkin JL, Kato BS, et al. The Association between Physical Activity in Leisure Time and Leukocyte Telomere Length. *Arch Intern Med*. Arch Intern Med.

[32] Shin YA, Lee JH, Song W, et al. Exercise Training Improves the Antioxidant Enzyme Activity with No Changes of Telomere Length. *Mech Ageing Dev*. 2008 May;129(5):254-60.

[33] Ornish D, Lin J, Daubenmier J, et al. Increased Telomerase Activity and Comprehensive Lifestyle Changes: A Pilot Study. *Lancet Oncol*. 2008 Nov;9(11):1048-57

[34] Pizzorno, Lara. Slowing Telomere Attrition and Cellular Senescence Today, Part II. Longevity Medicine Review. http://www.lmreview.com/

[35] Graham, Danielle. Genetics, Epigenetics and Destiny. An Interview With Bruce Lipton. http://www.superconsciousness.com

[36] Tarone, RE, Blot, WJ, McLaughlin, JK. Nonselective Nonaspirin Nonsteroidal Anti-Inflammatory Drugs and Gastrointestinal Bleeding: Relative and Absolute Risk Estimates from Recent Epidemiologic Studies. *Am J Ther* 2004;**11**(1):17–25.

[37] Singh, G, Triadafilopoulos, G. Epidemiology of NSAID Induced Gastrointestinal Complications. *J Rheumatol* 1999;**26**(suppl):18–24.

[38] Ames BN. Low Micronutrient Intake May Accelerate the Degenerative Diseases of Aging Through Allocation of Scarce Micronutrients by Triage. Proc. Natl. Acad. Sci. U.S.A. 2006;103:17589-94.

[39] ibid

[40] Biaglow JE, et al. Role of glutathione and other thiols in cellular response to radiation and drugs. *Drug Metab Rev* 1989;20:1-12.

[41] Aw TY. Intestinal Glutathione: Determinant of Mucosal Peroxide Transport, Metabolism, and Oxidative Susceptibility.
Toxicol Appl Pharmacol. 2005 May 1;204(3):320-8.

[42] Dvoráková M, Sivonová M, et al.   The Effect of Polyphenolic Extract from Pine Bark, Pycnogenol on the Level of
Glutathione in Children Suffering from Attention Deficit Hyperactivity Disorder (ADHD). Redox Rep. 2006;11(4):163-72.

[43] Li YJ, Scott WK, et al. Revealing the Role of Glutathione S-transferase Omega in Age-at-Onset of Alzheimer and Parkinson Diseases. Neurobiol Aging. 2006 Aug;27(8):1087-93. Epub 2005 Jun 27.

[44] Kaufmann Y, Todorova VK, Luo S, Klimberg VS. Glutamine Affects Glutathione Recycling Enzymes in a DMBA-Induced Breast Cancer Model. Nutr Cancer. 2008;60(4):518-25.

[45] Odom RY, Dansby MY, Rollins-Hairston AM, Jackson KM, Kirlin WG. Phytochemical Induction of Cell Cycle Arrest by Glutathione Oxidation and Reversal by N-acetylcysteine in Human Colon Carcinoma Cells. Nutr Cancer. 2009;61(3):332-9.

[46] Ji DB, Ye J, Li CL, Wang YH, Zhao J, Cai SQ. Antiaging Effect of Cordyceps Sinensis Extract. Phytother Res. 2009 Jan;23(1):116-22.

[47] Ames BN. Low Micronutrient Intake May Accelerate the Degenerative Diseases of Aging Through Allocation of Scarce Micronutrients by Triage. Proc. Natl. Acad. Sci. U.S.A. 2006;103:17589-94.

[48] Fenech M. The Role of Folic Acid and Vitamin B12 in Genomic Stability of Human Cells. *Mutat Res.* 2001 Apr 18;475(1-2):57-67.

[49] Ames BN, Elson-Schwab I, Silver EA. High-dose Vitamin Therapy Stimulate Variant Enzymes with Decreased Coenzyme-binding Affinity (increased Km): Relevance to Genetic Disease and Polymorphisms. Am. J. Clin. Nutr. 2002;75:616-58.

[50] Riedl, et al. Oral Sulforaphane Increases Phase II Antioxidant Enzymes in the Human Upper Airway. Clinical Immunology (2009) vol. 130 (3) pp. 244-251

[51] Albensi BC, Mattson MP (2000). "Evidence for the involvement of TNF and NF-κB in hippocampal synaptic plasticity". *Synapse* 35 (2): 151–9

[52] Brasier AR (2006). "The NF-κB Regulatory Network". *Cardiovasc. Toxicol.* 6 (2): 111–30.

[53] Bhagavan HN, Chopra RK. Coenzyme Q10: Absorption, Tissue Uptake, Metabolism and Pharmacokinetics. Free Radic Res. 2006 May;40(5):445-53.

[54] Yasko, Amy. Genetic Bypass, Using Nutrition to Bypass Genetic Mutations; Matrix Development Publishing, 2005.

[55] Yang XD, Tajkhorshid E, Chen LF. Functional Interplay Between Acetylation and Methylation of the RelA Subunit of NF-kappaB.
Mol Cell Biol. 2010 May;30(9):2170-80. Epub 2010 Feb 16.

[56] Vitamin B Supplements Could Delay Onset of Alzheimer's, Says Study.
http://www.guardian.co.uk/lifeandstyle/2010/sep/08/vitamin-b-could-delays-alzheimers

[57] Tonetti M, Sturia L, Bistolfi T, Benatti U, De Flora A. Extracellular ATP Potentiates Nitric Oxide
Synthase Expression Induced by Lipopolysaccharide in RAW 264.7 Murine Macrophages. Biochem
Biophys Res Commun. 1994:203(1):430-5.

[58] Mortensen DP, Gonzalez-Alonso J, Bune LT, et al. ATP-induced Vasodilation and Purinergic
Receptors in the Human Leg: Roles of Nitric Oxide, Prostaglandins and Adenosine. Am J Physiol
Regul Integr Comp Physiol. 2009;296:R1140-R1148.

[59] Bivalacqua TJ, Liu T, et al.   Endothelial Nitric Oxide Synthase Keeps Erection Regulatory Function Balance in
the Penis. Eur Urol. 2007 Jun;51(6):1732-40.

[60] Harris MB, Mitchell BM, et al. Increased Nitric Oxide Synthase Activity and Hsp90 Association in Skeletal Muscle
Following Chronic Exercise. Eur J Appl Physiol. 2008 Nov;104(5):795-802.

[61] Miljkovic D, Trajkovic V. Inducible Nitric Oxide Synthase Activation by Interleukin-17.
Cytokine Growth Factor Rev. 2004 Feb;15(1):21-32.

[62] Pall, Martin. Explaining "Unexplained Illnesses". Informa HealthCare; New York. 2009

[63] Sears, Barry. The Age-Free Zone.Haper Collins Books, NY, NY; 2000, p.162

[64] Ibid; p.167.

[65] Sartore G, Lapolla A, et al. Desaturase Activities and Metabolic Control in Type 2 Diabetes. Prostaglandins LeukotEssent Fatty Acids. 2008 Jul-Aug;79(1-2):55-8.

[66] Reese AC, Fradet V, Witte JS. Omega-3 Fatty Acids, Genetic Variants in COX-2 and Prostate Cancer.J NutrigenetNutrigenomics. 2009;2(3):149-58.

[67] Simopolous, Artemis. Essential Fatty Acids in Health and Chronic Disease. The American Journal of Clinical Nutrition, Vol 70, No. 3, 5605-5695, September, 1999.

[68] Lipton, Bruce, The Biology of Belief. Hay House Inc. 2005

[69] Weitz D, et al. Fish Oil for the Treatment of Cardiovascular Disease. *Cardiol Rev. 2010 Sep-Oct;18(5):258-63.*

[70] Di Minno MN, et al. Exploring Newer CardioprotectiveSstrategies: Omega-3 Fatty Acids in Perspective. *ThrombHaemost. 2010 Aug 30;104(4).*

[71] Endres S, Ghorbany R, Kelley V *et al.* The Effect of Dietary Supplementation With n-3 Polyunsaturated Fatty Acids on the Synthesis of Interleukin-1 and Tumor Necrosis Factor by Mononuclear Cells. N Engl J Med 1989; 320: 265–71.

[72] Meydani S, Endres S, Wood M *et al.* Oral n-3 Fatty Acid Supplementation Suppresses Cytokine Production and Lymphocyte Proliferation. Comparison in Young and Older Women. J Nutr 1991; 121: 547–55.

[73] Barham JB, Edens MB, Fonteh AN, Johnson MM, Easter L, Chilton FH (August 2000). "Addition of Eicosapentaenoic Acid to Gamma-Linolenic Acid-Supplemented Diets Prevents Serum Arachidonic Acid Accumulation in Humans". *J. Nutr.*130 (8): 1925–31.

[74] Johnson MM, Swan DD, Surette ME, *et al.* (1997). "Dietary Supplementation With γ-Linolenic Acid Alters Fatty Acid Content and Eicosanoid Production in Healthy Humans"*J. Nutr.*127 (8): 1435–44.

[75] Mozaffarian D, Katan MB, Ascherio A, Stampfer MJ, Willett WC.Trans Fatty Acids and Cardiovascular Disease. *N Engl J Med.* 2006; 354:1601-13.

[76] Willett WC, Stampfer MJ, Manson JE, et al. Intake of Trans Fatty Acids and Risk of Coronary Heart Disease Among Women. *Lancet.*1993; 341:581-585.

[77] Matthias, B. and Schulze, M.B. Dietary Pattern, Inflammation, and Incidence of Type 2 Diabetes in Women. Am J ClinNutr.Sep 2005; 82: 675-684.

[78] Heaton, K. The Sweet Road to Gallstones. Brit Med J. Apr 14, 1984; 288: 1103-1104.

[79] Welsh et al., Caloric Sweetener Consumption and Dyslipidemia Among US Adults, JAMA, April 2010, 303(15)

[80] Yudkin, J. Sugar Consumption and Myocardial Infarction. Lancet. Feb 6, 1971; 1(7693): 296-297.

[81] Profiling Food Consumption in America. http://www.usda.gov/factbook/chapter2.pdf

[82] Enig, Mary G, PhD, *Trans Fatty Acids in the Food Supply: A Comprehensive Report Covering 60 Years of Research*, 2nd Edition, Enig Associates, Inc, Silver Spring, MD, 1995, 4-8

[83] Fernandez, N A, *Cancer Res*, 1975, 35:3272; Martines, I, et al, Cancer Res, 1975, 35:3265

[84] Pitskhelauri, G Z, *The Long Living of Soviet Georgia*, 1982, Human Sciences Press, New York, NY

[85] Koga, Y et al, "Recent Trends in Cardiovascular Disease and Risk Factors in the Seven Countries Study: Japan," *Lessons for Science from the Seven Countries Study*, H Toshima, et al, eds, Springer, New York, NY, 1994, 63-74

[86] Moore, Thomas J, *Lifespan: What Really Affects Human Longevity*, 1990, Simon and Schuster, New York, NY

[87] Enig, Mary G, Ph D, et al, *Fed Proc*, Jul 1978, 37:9:2215-2220

[88] Ausubel, Kenny. *When Healing Becomes a Crime*; Rochester, VT: Healing Arts Press, 2000, p. 118

[89] Cuthbert S, Rosner A, Technique Summary: Applied Kinesiology: http://www.chiroaccess.com/Articles/Technique-Summary-Applied-Kinesiology.aspx?id=0000144

[90] What Is AK?: http://www.icakusa.com

[91] Types of Kinesiology: http://www.kinesiologyshop.com

[92] Schmitt, Walter; http://www.theuplink.com

[93] Astil-Smith, Chris; http://www.metabolics.com

[94] Lebowitz, Michael; http://www.michaellebowitzdc.com

[95] Schmitt, Walter H., Yanuck, Samuel; Expanding the Neurological Examination Using Functional Neurologic Assessment: Part I, The Neurologic Basis of Applied Kinesiology. International Journal of Neuroscience, vol 97. Issue 1 &2. March 1999. pp. 77-108

[96] Cuthbert SC, Goodheart GJ Jr., On The Reliability and Validity of Manual Muscle Testing: A Literature Review, *Chiropr Osteopat.* 2007 Mar 6;15(1):4.

[97] Walther, David; Applied Kinesiology Synopsis, 2nd edition. Systems DC, 2000, p. 347

[98] Reeves & Swenson, Disorders of the Nervous System, http://www.dartmouth.edu/ ~dons/part_1/chapter_8.html#chpt_8

[99] Monrad-Krohn, G.H., Refsum S.: The Clinical Examination of the Nervous System, ed. 12, London, H.K. Lewis & Co., 1964.

[100] DeJong, R.N.: The Neurologic Examination, ed. 4. New York, Paul B. Hoeber, Inc., 1958.

[101] Wartenberg, R.: The Examination of Reflexes: A Simplification. Chicago, Year book Medical Publishers, 1945.

[102] Woolf CJ, Ma Q. Nociceptors—Noxious Stimulus Detectors. Neuron. 2007 Aug 2;55(3):353-64. Review. PubMed PMID: 17678850.

[103] K Jensen et al., The Lancet Nov 8 1975, p.920

[104] Stephens JA, Reinking RM, Stuart DG (1975) J Neurophysiology 38:1217-1231

[105] Miller, Herbert, The Role of Autogenic Inhibition in the Reduction of Muscle Splinting. http://www.ncbi.nlm.nih.gov/pmc/articles/PMC2484598/

[106] Sympathetic Outflow Enhances the Stretch Reflex Response in the Relaxed Soleus Muscle in Humans. *J Appl Physiol* 98: 1366-1370, 2005.

[107] McCulloch M, Jezierski T, et al. Diagnostic Accuracy of Canine Scent Detection in Early- and Late-Stage Lung and Breast Cancers. Integr Cancer Ther. 2006 Mar;5(1):30-9.

[108] Machado RF, Laskowski D, et al. Detection of Lung Cancer by Sensor Array Analyses of Exhaled Breath. Am J Respir Crit Care Med. 2005 Jun 1;171(11):1286-91.

[109] Bajtarevic A, Ager C, et al. Noninvasive Detection of Lung Cancer by Analysis of Exhaled Breath. BMC Cancer. 2009 Sep 29;9:348.

[110] Horvath G, Järverud GA, et al. Human Ovarian Carcinomas Detected by Specific Odor. Integr Cancer Ther. 2008 Jun;7(2):76-80.

[111] Sonoda H, Kohnoe S, et al. Colorectal Cancer Screening with Odour Material by Canine Scent Detection. Gut. 2011 Jan 31. [Epub ahead of print]

[112] Guyton, Arthur C. &Hall, John E., Textbook of Medical Physiology, 11th Edition; Saunders Publishing, 2005

[113] Guyton, Arthur C. Textbook of Medical Physiology. W.B. Saunders Co, 8th ed. 1991. p. 29

[114] Electron, Wikipedia.org, http://en.wikipedia.org/wiki/Electrons#cite_note-de_broglie-47

[115] Atom, Wikipedia.org, http://en.wikipedia.org/wiki/Atom

[116] Electromagnetic Waves, Univ of Waterloo, http://science.uwaterloo.ca/~cchieh/cact//c120/emwave.html

[117] Becker, Richard. Electromagnetic Fields and Interactions; Blaisdell Publishing, 1982, p. 59

[118] Edwards, J.C. "Principles of NMR." Process NMR Associates: http://www.process-nmr.com/pdfs/NMR%20Overview.pdf. Retrieved 2009-02-23.

[119] Keeler, James. Understanding NMR Spectroscopy: http://www-keeler.ch.cam.ac.uk/lectures/Irvine/chapter2.pdf.

[120] Choices in Testing for Complete Cardiovascular Care, http://www.labcorp.com/pdf/Cardiovascular_flyer_L4719_0407_1.pdf

[121] Otvos JD. Measurement of Lipoprotein Subclass Profiles by Nuclear Magnetic Resonance Spectroscopy. In: Rifai N, Warnick GR, Dominiczak MH, eds. Handbook of Lipoprotein Testing. 2nd ed. Washington DC: AACC Press; 2000:609-623.

[122] Otvos J, Jeyarajah E, Bennett D. A Spectroscopic Approach to Lipoprotein Subclass Analysis. J Clin Ligand Assay. 1996; 19(3):184-189.

[123] Dolphin, Lambert: http://ldolphin.org/light.html

[124] D'Adamo, Peter J. Live Right 4 Your Type, Penguin Putnam Inc. New York, 2001. p. 4

[125] Guyton, Arthur C. & Hall, John E., Textbook of Medical Physiology, 11th Edition; Saunders Publishing, 2005

[126] Pressman AS, Electromagnetic Fields and Life; Plenum Press, New York 1970

[127] Dubrov AP, The Geomagnetic Field and Life: Geomagneticbiology; Plenum Press, New York, 1978

[128] Ho M W, The Rainbow and the Worm: The Physics of Organism, 2nd ed. World Scientific, River Edge, NJ 1998

[129] Marino, A.A. & Carrubba, S. The Effects of Mobile-Phone Electromagnetic Fields on Brain Electrical nd Activity: A Critical Analysis of the Literature. Med. Biol. 28:250–274, 2009.

[130] Kheifets L, Shimkhada R. Childhood Leukemia and EMF: Review of the Epidemiologic Evidence. Bioelectromagnetics. 2005;Suppl 7:S51-9.

[131] Brainard GC, Kavet R, Kheifets LI. The Relationship Between Electromagnetic Field and Light Exposures to Melatonin and Breast Cancer Risk: A Review of the Relevant Literature. J Pineal Res. 1999 Mar;26(2):65-100.

[132] Oschman, James L, Energy Medicine: The Scientific Basis, Churchill Livingstone, 2000 p.176

[133] Ibid

[134] Adey W R, Balwin S M, Brain Interactions with Weak Electric and Magnetic Fields; Neurosciences Research Program Bulletin, 1997 15(1):1-129

[135] Adey W R, Electromagnetic Fields and the Essence of Living Systems: Modern Radio Science. Oxford University Press, Oxford 1990 pp. 1-36

[136] Seasonal Affective Disorder, The Mayo Clinic.org, http://www.mayoclinic.com/health/seasonal-affective-disorder/DS00195

[137] Miller AL., Epidemiology, Etiology, and Natural Treatment of Seasonal Affective Disorder. Altern Med Rev. 2005 Mar;10(1):5-13.

[138] Hirota T, Fukada Y., Resetting Mechanism of Central and Peripheral Circadian Clocks in Mammals. Zoolog Sci. 2004 Apr;21(4):359-68.

[139] Holick MF. Vitamin D: Importance in the Prevention of Cancers, Type 1 Diabetes, Heart Disease, and Osteoporosis. Am J Clin Nutr. 2004 Mar;79(3):362-71.

[140] Chowdhury I, Sengupta A, Maitra SK., Melatonin: Fifty Years of Scientific Journey From the Discovery in Bovine Pineal Gland to Delineation of Functions in Humans. Indian J Biochem Biophys. 2008 Oct;45(5):289-304.

[141] Holick MF., Photosynthesis of Vitamin D in the Skin: Effect of Environmental and Life-style Variables. Fed Proc. 1987 Apr;46(5):1876-82.

[142] Campbell SS, Murphy PJ., Extraocular Circadian Phototransduction in Humans. Science. 1998 Jan 16;279(5349):396-9.

[143] Oschman, James L, Energy Medicine: The Scientific Basis, Churchill Livingstone, 2000 p.179-181

[144] Ibid

[145] The Bird's Sixth Sense: How They See Magnetic Fields. http://blogs.discovermagazine.com/80beats/2009/10/29/the-birds-sixth-sense-how-they-see-magnetic-fields/

[146] Oschman, James L, Energy Medicine: The Scientific Basis, Churchill Livingstone, 2000 p.45

[147] Busse JW, Bhandari M, Kulkarni AV, Tunks E., The Effect of Low-intensity Pulsed Ultrasound Therapy on Time to Fracture Healing: A Meta-analysis. CMAJ. 2002 Feb 19;166(4):437-41.

[148] Bedwell C, Dowswell T, Neilson JP, Lavender T., The use of Transcutaneous Electrical Nerve Stimulation (TENS) for Pain Relief in Labour: A Review of the Evidence. Midwifery. 2010 Feb 17.

[149] Eichler , David, A. Study of a Subtle Energy Transduction Device on Anxiety Levels of Students in a Public School Setting. Journal of Alternative & Complementary Medicine: RUBIK/SRT& trade PAPER, Vol. 8, #6 (pp 823-856)

[150] National Center for Health Statistics, http://www.cdc.gov/nchs/FASTATS/lcod.htm

[151] Starfield B, Is US Health Really the Best in the World?, (JAMA), July 26th, 2000, vol. 284, No. 4

[152] Brodie, Douglas, Cancer and Common Sense, Combining Science and Nature to Control Cancer. Winning Publications. White Bear Lake, MN 1997.

[153] Diamond J, Cowden L, Goldberg J, An Alternative Medicine Definitive Guide to Cancer. Future Medicine Publishing. Tiburon, CA 1997.

[154] Smith, Ben et al, Journal of Clinical Oncology, April 29, 2009; University of Texas M.D. Cancer Center.

[155] National Center for Health Statistics, http://www.cdc.gov/nchs/FASTATS/lcod.htm

[156] Bottorff MB., Am J Cardiol. Statin Safety and Drug Interactions: Clinical Implications. 2006 Apr 17;97(8A):27C-31C.

[157] Tirkkonen T, Ryynänen A, Vahlberg T, Irjala K, Klaukka T, Huupponen R, Laine K. Frequency and Clinical Relevance of Drug Interactions with Lovastatin and Simvastatin: An Observational Database Study; Drug Saf. 2008;31(3):231-40.

[158] Roberts DJ, Pain A, Kai O, Kortok M, Marsh K. Lancet. Autoagglutination of Malaria-infected Red Blood Cells and Malaria Severity. 2000 Apr 22;355(9213):1427-8.

[159] Shill HA, Alaedini A, et al. Anti-ganglioside Antibodies in Idiopathic and Hereditary Cerebellar Degeneration. Neurology. 2003 May 27;60(10):1672-3.

[160] Humphrey LL, Fu R, Rogers K, Freeman M, Helfand M. Homocysteine Level and Coronary Heart Disease Incidence: A Systematic Review and Meta-analysis. Mayo Clin Proc. 2008 Nov;83(11):1203-12.

[161] Jamison RL, Hartigan P et al. Effect of Homocysteine Lowering on Mortality and Vascular Disease in Advanced Chronic Kidney Disease and End-stage Renal Disease: A Randomized Controlled Trial. JAMA. 2007 Sep 12;298(10):1163-70.

[162] Humphrey LL, Fu R, Rogers K, Freeman M, Helfand M. Homocysteine Level and Coronary Heart Disease Incidence: A Systematic Review and Meta-analysis. Mayo Clin Proc. 2008 Nov;83(11):1203-12.

[163] Heinz J, Kropf S, Luley C, Dierkes. Homocysteine as A Risk Factor for Cardiovascular Disease in Patients Treated by Dialysis: A Meta-analysis. J. Am J Kidney Dis. 2009 Sep;54(3):478-89.

[164] Yasko, Amy. Genetic Bypass, Using Nutrition to Bypass Genetic Mutations; Matrix Development Publishing, 2005.

[165] Ferreira PC, Piai Kde A, et al. Aluminum as a Risk Factor for Alzheimer's Disease. Rev Lat Am Enfermagem. 2008 Jan-Feb;16(1):151-7.

[166] Perl DP, Good PF. The Association of Aluminum Alzheimer's Disease, and Neurofibrillary Tangles. J Neural Transm Suppl. 1987;24:205-11.

[167] Miu AC, Benga O. Aluminum and Alzheimer's Disease: A New Look. J Alzheimers Dis. 2006 Nov;10(2-3):179-201.

[168] Faesch S, Jennane F et al. Thyroiditis and Gluten Intolerance: Extrapancreatic Auto-immune Diseases Associated with Type 1 Diabetes. Arch Pediatr. 2007 Jan;14(1):24-30.

[169] Ivarsson A, Persson LA, et al. Epidemic of Coeliac Disease in Swedish Children. Acta Paediatr. 2000 Feb;89(2):165-71.

[170] Ivarsson A, Persson LA, Hernell O. Does Breast-feeding Affect the Risk for Coeliac Disease? Adv Exp Med Biol. 2000;478:139-49.

[171] Weile B, Krasilnikoff PA. Extremely Low Incidence Rates of Celiac Disease in the Danish Population of Children. J Clin Epidemiol. 1993 Jul;46(7):661-4.

[172] Agranoff BW, and Goldberg D. Diet and the Geographical Distribution of Multiple Sclerosis. Lancet 2(7888) (November 2 1974): 1061-1066.

[173] Malosse D, Perron H, Sasco A, Seigneurin JM. Correlation Between Milk and Dairy Product Consumption and Multiple Sclerosis Prevalence: A Worldwide Study. Neuroepidemiology. 1992;11(4-6):304-12.

[174] Akerblom HK, Vaarala O, Hyoty H, et al. "Environmental Factors in the Etiology of Type I Diabetes." Am. J. Med. Genet. (Semin. Med. Genet.) 115 (2002): 18-29.

[175] Larsson SC, Andersson SO, Johansson JE, Wolk A. Cultured Milk, Yogurt, and Dairy Intake in Relation to Bladder Cancer Risk in a Prospective Study of Swedish Women and Men. Am J Clin Nutr. 2008 Oct;88(4):1083-7.

[176] Larsson SC, Bergkvist L, et al. Calcium and Dairy Food Intakes are Inversely Associated with Colorectal Cancer Risk in the Cohort of Swedish Men. Am J Clin Nutr. 2006 Mar;83(3):667-73; quiz 728-9.

[177] Naghma Khan, Farrukh Afaq and Hasan Mukhtar. Apoptosis by Dietary Factors: The Suicide Solution for Delaying Cancer Growth. Department of Dermatology, University of Wisconsin–Madison, Medical Sciences Center B-25, 1300 University Avenue, Madison, WI 53706, USA

[178] McCullough ML, Rodriguez C, Diver WR, Feigelson HS, Stevens VL, Thun MJ, Calle EE. Dairy, Calcium, and Vitamin D Intake and Postmenopausal Breast Cancer Risk in the Cancer Prevention Study II Nutrition Cohort. Cancer Epidemiol Biomarkers Prev. 2005 Dec;14(12):2898-904.

[179] Ames, Bruce. Low Micronutrient Intake May Accelerate the Degenerative Diseases of Aging Through Allocation of Scarce Micronutrients by Triage. Proc Natl Acad Sci U S A. 2006 November 21; 103(47): 17589–17594.

[180] Cox IM, Campbell MJ, Dawson D: Red Cell Magnesium and Chronic Fatigue Syndrome. Lancet 337:757, 1991

[181] Lodi R, Iotti S, Cortelli P, Pierangeli G, Cevoli S, Clementi V, Soriani S, Montagna P, Barbiroli B.: Deficient Energy Metabolism is Associated with Low Free Magnesium in the Brains of Patients with Migraine and Cluster Headache. Brain Res Bull. 2001 Mar 1;54(4):437-41.

[182] Van Houdenhove B, Pae CU, Luyten P: Chronic Fatigue Syndrome: Is There a Role for Non-antidepressant pharmacotherapy? Expert Opinion Pharmacotherapy. 2010 Feb;11(2):215-23.

[183] Ho E, Courtemanche C, Ames BN. Zinc Deficiency Induces Oxidative DNA Damage and Increases P53 Expression in Human Lung Fibroblasts. J. Nutr. 2003;133:2543-8.

[184] Lebbink JH, Fish A, Reumer A, Natrajan G, Winterwerp HH, Sixma TK: Magnesium Coordination Controls the Molecular Switch Function of DNA Mismatch Repair Protein Mutations. J Biol Chem. 2010 Feb 18.

[185] Ames, BN, JH Suh and J Lui. Enzymes Lose Binding Affinity (increased K_m) for Coenzymes and Substrates with Age: A Strategy for Remediation. 2006. *Nutrigenomics: Discovering the Path to Personalized Nutrition*, John Wiley & Sons, New Jersey, pp. 277-94

[186] Kaput, J. 2006. Diet – Disease Interactions at the Molecular Level: An Experimental Paradigm. *Phytochemicals: Nutrient–Gene Interactions.* M. Meskin, Bidlack, WR, and Randoph, RK. (Ed.) CRC Press. Pg 23 – 39.

[187] Wu Y, Liu Y, Han Y, et al. Pyridoxine Increases Nitric Oxide Biosynthesis in Human Platelets. Int J Vitam Nutr Res. 2009 Mar;79(2):95-103.

[188] Schmidt DR, Holmstrom SR, Fon Tacer K, et al: Regulation of Bile Acid Synthesis by Fat-soluble Vitamins A and D. J Biol Chem. 2010 Mar 16.

[189] Maczurek A, Hager K, Kenklies M, et al: Lipoic Acid as an Anti-inflammatory and Neuroprotective Treatment for Alzheimer's Disease. Adv Drug Deliv Rev. 2008 Oct-Nov;60(13-14):1463-70.

[190] Dimeloe S, Nanzer A, Ryanna K, Hawrylowicz C.J, Regulatory T Cells, Inflammation and the Allergic response-The Role of Glucocorticoids and Vitamin D. Steroid Biochem Mol Biol. 2010 Mar 18.

[191] Gorman C, Park A, Del K, Health: The Fires Within. Time Magazine; Feb, 2004;161:8

[192] Falder S, Silla R, Phillips M, Rea S, et al., Thiamine Supplementation Increases Serum Thiamine and Reduces Pyruvate and Lactate Levels in Burn Patients. Burns. 2010 Mar;36(2):261-9.

[193] Jiang Q, Ames BN. γ-Tocopherol, But Not α-tocopherol, Decreases Proinflammatory Eicosanoids and Inflammation Damage in Rats. FASEB J. 2003;17:816-22.

[194] Bolander FF., Vitamins: Not Just for Enzymes. Curr Opin Investig Drugs. 2006 Oct;7(10):912-5.

[195] Shay KP, Moreau RF, Smith EJ, Smith AR, Hagen TM: Alpha-lipoic Acid as a Dietary Supplement: Molecular Mechanisms and Therapeutic Potential. Biochim Biophys Acta. 2009 Oct;1790(10):1149-60.

[196] García OP, Long KZ, Rosado JL., Impact of Micronutrient Deficiencies on Obesity. Nutr Rev. 2009 Oct;67(10):559-72.

[197] Major GC, Alarie F, Doré J, Phouttama S, Tremblay A: Supplementation with Calcium + Vitamin D Enhances the Beneficial Effect of Weight Loss on Plasma Lipid and Lipoprotein Concentrations. Am J Clin Nutr. 2007 Jan;85(1):54-9.

[198] Plaisance EP, Lukasova M: Niacin Stimulates Adiponectin Secretion Through the GPR109A Receptor. Am J Physiol Endocrinol Metab. 2009 Mar;296(3):E549-58.

[199] Hatzitolios A, Iliadis F, Katsiki N, Baltatzi M.: Is the Anti-hypertensive Effect of Dietary Supplements Via Aldehydes Reduction Evidence Based? A Systematic Review. Clin Exp Hypertens. 2008 Oct;30(7):628-39.

[200] Houston MC.: Treatment of Hypertension with Nutraceuticals, Vitamins, Antioxidants and Minerals. Expert Rev Cardiovasc Ther. 2007 Jul;5(4):681-91.

[201] Wilburn AJ, King DS, Glisson J, Rockhold RW, Wofford MR.: The Natural Teatment of Hypertension. J Clin Hypertens (Greenwich). 2004 May;6(5):242-8.

[202] Kendler BS: Supplemental Conditionally Essential Nutrients in Cardiovascular Disease Therapy. J Cardiovasc Nurs. 2006 Jan-Feb;21(1):9-16.

[203] Eby GA 3rd, Eby KL., Magnesium for Treatment-resistant Depression: A Review and Hypothesis., Med Hypotheses. 2010 Apr;74(4):649-60.

[204] Dodig-Curković K, Dovhanj J, et al: The Role of Zinc in the Treatment of Hyperactivity Disorder in Children. Acta Med Croatica. 2009 Oct;63(4):307-13.

[205] Fava M, Mischoulon D: Folate in Depression: Efficacy, Safety, Differences in Formulations, and Clinical Issues. J Clin Psychiatry. 2009;70 Suppl 5:12-7.

[206] Bolander FF., Vitamins: Not Just for Enzymes. Curr Opin Investig Drugs. 2006 Oct;7(10):912-5.

[207] Yamaguchi M., Role of Nutritional Zinc in the Prevention of Osteoporosis. Mol Cell Biochem. 2009 Dec 25.

[208] Ames BN. Low Micronutrient Intake May Accelerate the Degenerative Diseases of Aging Through Allocation of Scarce Micronutrients by Triage. Proc. Natl. Acad. Sci. U.S.A. 2006;103:17589-94.

[209] Spellacy WN, Buhi WC, Birk SA.: Vitamin B6 Treatment of Gestational Diabetes Mellitus: Studies of Blood Glucose and Plasma Insulin. Am J Obstet Gynecol. 1977 Mar 15;127(6):599-602.

[210] Rosenblatt J, Bissonnette A, Ahmad R, Wu Z, Vasir B, et al: Immunomodulatory Effects of Vitamin D: Implications for GVHD. Bone Marrow Transplant. 2010 Jan 18.

[211] Killilea DW, Maier JA. A Connection Between Magnesium Deficiency and Aging: New Insights From Cellular Studies. *Magnes Res*. 2008 Jun;21(2):77-82.

[212] Killilea DW, Ames BN. Magnesium Deficiency Accelerates Cellular Senescence in Cultured Human Fibroblasts. *Proc Natl Acad Sci* U S A. 2008 Apr 15;105(15):5768-73.

[213] Ranieri M, Sciuscio M, Cortese AM, et al: The Use of Alpha-lipoic Acid (ALA), Gamma Linolenic Acid (GLA) and Rehabilitation in the Treatment of Back Pain: Effect on Health-related Quality of Life. Int J Immunopathol Pharmacol. 2009 Jul-Sep;22(3 Suppl):45-50.

[214] Rosenberg EI, Genao I, Chen I, et al: Complementary and Alternative Medicine Use by Primary Care Patients with Chronic Pain. Pain Med. 2008 Nov;9(8):1065-72.

[215] Bertollo CM, Oliveira AC: Characterization of the Antinociceptive and Anti-inflammatory Activities of Riboflavin in Different Experimental Models. Eur J Pharmacol. 2006 Oct 10;547(1-3):184-91.

[216] Ames BN. Low Micronutrient Intake May Accelerate the Degenerative Diseases of Aging Through Allocation of Scarce Micronutrients by Triage. Proc. Natl. Acad. Sci. U.S.A. 2006;103:17589-94.

[217] Ames BN, Elson-Schwab I, Silver EA. High-dose Vitamin Therapy Stimulate Variant Enzymes with Decreased Coenzyme-binding Affinity (increased Km): Relevance to Genetic Disease and Polymorphisms. Am. J. Clin. Nutr. 2002;75:616-58.

[218] Flegal K, Carroll M, et al. Prevalence and Trends in Obesity Among US Adults, 1999-2008. JAMA. 2010;303(3):235-241.

[219] http://www.ers.usda.gov/publications/foodreview/sep1996/ sept96d.pdf

[220] Cannon C, Elizabeth V, The Complete Idiots Guide to the Anti-Inflammation Diet. Penguin Books, 2006; p. 160

[221] Thiel RJ. Natural Vitamins May be Superior to Synthetic Ones. Med Hypotheses. 2000 Dec;55(6):461-9.

[222] Han SN, Pang E, et al. Differential Effects of Natural and Synthetic Vitamin E on Gene Transcription in Murine T Lymphocytes. Arch Biochem Biophys. 2010 Mar 1;495(1):49-55.

[223] Smith J, Seeds of Deception. Yes Books, Fairfiled, Iowa. 2003: p. 48

[224] Setnikar I, Giacchetti C, and Zanolo G. Pharmacokinetics of Glucosamine. *Drug Res* 1986; 36:729-734.

[225] D'Ambrosio E, Casa B, Bompani R, Scali G, Scali M. Glucosamine Sulfate: A Controlled Clinical Investigation in Arthrosis. Pharmacotherapeutica 1981; 2(8):504-508.

[226] Drovanti A, Bignamini AA, Rovati AL. Therapeutic Activity of Oral Glucosamine Sulfate in Osteoarthrosis: A Placebo-controlled Double-blind Investigation. *Clin Ther* 1998; 3:260-272.

[227] Dickenson, Annette, Who Uses Vitamin and Mineral Supplements?, http://www.crnusa.org/benpdfs/CRN011benefits_whovms.pdf

[228] Adebowale A, Cox D, et al. Analysis of Glucosamine and Chondroitin Sulfate Content in Marketed Products, http://www.ana-jana.org/reprints/EddingtonStudy.pdf

[229] Beal B. "Evaluation of Active Enzyme Activity in Six Oral Superoxide Dismutase Products." Paper presented at the 25th Annual Conference of the Veterinary Orthopedic Society, Snowmass, Colorado, 1998;65.

[230] Moore T. Messing with Mother Nature. *The Washingtonian* July 1999; 58-115.

[231] Li Y, Wang C, Zhu K, Feng RN, Sun CH., Effects of Multivitamin and Mineral Supplementation on Adiposity, Energy Expenditure and Lipid Profiles in Obese Chinese Women. Int J Obes (Lond). Feb 9, 2010.

[232] Taylor SI, Kadowaki T et al. Mutations in Insulin-Receptor Gene in Insulin-Resistant Patients. Diabetes Care. 1990 Mar;13(3):257-79.

[233] Suzuki Y, Hatanaka Y, et al. Insulin Resistance Associated With Decreased Levels of Insulin-Receptor Messenger Ribonucleic Acid: Evidence of a De Novo Mutation in the Maternal Allele. J Clin Endocrinol Metab. 1995 Apr;80(4):1214-20.

[234] The Relation of Salivary Cortisol to Patterns of Performance on a Word List Learning Task in Healthy Older Adults. Psycho Nuero Endo. 2008 Oct;33(9):1293-6

[235] Circadian Stage-Dependent Inhibition of Human Breast Cancer Metabolism and Growth by the Nocturnal Melatonin Signal: Consequences of Its Disruption by Light at Night in Rats and Women. Integr Cancer Ther. 2009 Dec;8(4):347-53

[236] Circadian Clock and Vascular Disease. Hypertens Res. 2010 May 7.

[237] Melatonin-Insulin Interactions in Patients with Metabolic Syndrome. J Pineal Res. 2008 Jan;44(1):52-6.

[238] Circadian Misalignment in Mood Disturbances. Curr Psychiatry Rep. 2009 Dec;11(6):459-65.

[239] Juvenile Diabetes Research Foundation. http://www.jdrfrockymountain.org/

[240] Chong JW, Craig ME, et al. Marked Increase in Type 1 Diabetes Mellitus Incidence in Children Aged 0-14 in Victoria, Australia, from 1999 to 2002. Pediatr Diabetes. 2007 Apr;8(2):67-73.

[241] Vitale C, Marazzi G et al. Metabolic Syndrome. Minerva Med. 2006 Jun;97(3):219-29.

[242] About Metabolic Syndrome. http://www.heart.org/HEARTORG/Conditions/More/MetabolicSyndrome/About-Metabolic-Syndrome_UCM_301920_Article.jsp

[243] Okinawa Centenarian Study. http://www.okicent.org/

[244] New England Centenarian Study. http://www.bumc.bu.edu/centenarian/

[245] Rosenthal M, Glew R. Medical Biochemistry: Human Metabolism in Health and Disease. John Wiley & Sons Publishing: 2009; p. 126

[246] Merrill AH Jr, Henderson JM. Vitamin B6 Metabolism by Human Liver. Ann N Y Acad Sci. 1990;585:110-7.

[247] Brownstein, David. Overcoming Thyroid Disorders. Medical Alternative Press, West Bloomfield MI, 2004. P. 196

[248] Keniston RC, Nathan PA, Leklem JE, Lockwood RS. Vitamin B6, Vitamin C, and Carpal Tunnel Syndrome. A Cross-Sectional Study of 441 Adults. J Occup Environ Med. 1997 Oct;39(10):949-59.

[249] Wang HS, Kuo MF et al. Pyridoxal Phosphate is Better than Pyridoxine for Controlling Idiopathic Intractable Epilepsy. Arch Dis Child. 2005 May;90(5):512-5.

[250] Wang YQ, Yao MH. J Nutr Biochem. Effects of Chromium Picolinate on Glucose Uptake in Insulin-Resistant 3T3-L1 Adipocytes Involve Activation of P38 MAPK. 2009 Dec;20(12):982-91.

[251] Zeyda M, Stulnig TM. Obesity, Inflammation, and Insulin Resistance—a Mini-Review. Gerontology. 2009;55(4):379-86.

[252] Sears, Barry. The Age-Free Zone. Haper Collins Books, NY, NY; 2000

[253] Zeyda M, Stulnig TM. Obesity, Inflammation, and Insulin Resistance—a Mini-Review. Gerontology. 2009;55(4):379-86.

[254] Giovannucci E. Metabolic Syndrome, Hyperinsulinemia, and Colon Cancer: A Review. Am J Clin Nutr. 2007 Sep;86(3):s836-42.

[255] Fujita T. Mineralocorticoid Receptors, Salt-Sensitive Hypertension, and Metabolic Syndrome. Hypertension. 2010 Apr;55(4):813-8.

[256] Chei CL, Yamagishi K et al. Metabolic Syndrome and the Risk of Ischemic Heart Disease and Stroke among Middle-Aged Japanese. Hypertens Res. 2008 Oct;31(10):1887-94.

[257] Fletcher, Kristin. Ten Most Common Health Complaints. http://www.forbes.com/2003/07/15/cx_kf_0715health.html

[258] Sandyk R. L-tryptophan in Neuropsychiatric Disorders: A Review. Int J Neurosci. 1992 Nov-Dec;67(1-4):127-44.

[259] Szabo, Liz. The Number of Americans Taking Antidepressants Doubles. USA Today, 2009

[260]Ostrow, Nicole http://www.bloomberg.com/apps/news, nostrow1@bloomberg.net.

[261] Kubera M, Lin AH, Kenis G, Bosmans E, van Bockstaele D, Maes M. "Anti-Inflammatory Effects of Antidepressants Through Suppression of the Interferon-Gamma/Interleukin-10 Production Ratio." J Clin Psychopharmacol. 2001 Apr;21(2):199-206

[262] Maes M."The Immunoregulatory Effects of Antidepressants." Hum Psychopharmacol. 2001 Jan;16(1):95-103

[263] Ferguson JM. The Effects of Antidepressants on Sexual Functioning in Depressed Patients: A Review. J Clin Psychiatry. 2001;62 Suppl 3:22-34.

[264] Cougnard A, Verdoux H, Grolleau A, Moride Y, Begaud B, Tournier M. Impact of Antidepressants on the Risk of Suicide in Patients with Depression In Real-life Conditions: A Decision Analysis Model. Psychol Med. 2009 Aug;39(8):1307-15.

[265] Exercise Found Effective Against Depression. http://www.nytimes.com/2000/10/10/health/exercise-found-effective-against-depression.html

[266] Caspi A, Sugden K, et al. Influence of Life Stress on Depression: Moderation by a Polymorphism in the 5-HTT Gene. Science. 2003 Jul 18;301(5631):386-9.

[267] Schroeder M, Krebs MO, et al. Epigenetics and Depression: Current Challenges and New Therapeutic Options. Curr Opin Psychiatry. 2010 Jul 16.

[268] Ancoli-Israel S, Roth T. Characteristics of Insomnia in the United States: Results of the 1991 National Sleep Foundation Survey. Sleep. 1999 May 1;22 Suppl 2:S347-53.

[269] Blask DE. Melatonin, Sleep Disturbance and Cancer Risk. Sleep Med Rev. 2009 Aug;13(4):257-64.

[270] Viswanathan AN, Schernhammer ES. Circulating Melatonin and the Risk of Breast and Endometrial Cancer in Women. Cancer Lett. 2009 Aug 18;281(1):1-7.

[271] Carrillo-Vico A, Guerrero JM, et al. A Review of the Multiple Actions of Melatonin on the Immune System. Endocrine. 2005 Jul;27(2):189-200.

[272] Szczepanik M. Melatonin and Its Influence on the Immune System. J Physiol Pharmacol. 2007 Dec;58 Suppl 6:115-24.

[273] Wu YH, Swaab DF. The Human Pineal Gland and Melatonin in Aging and Alzheimer's Disease. J Pineal Res. 2005 Apr;38(3):145-52.

[274] Král' A. The Role of Pineal Gland in Circadian Rhythm Regulation. Bratisl Lek Listy. 1994 Jul;95(7):295-303.

[275] Wiley TS, Lights Out, Sleep Sugar and Survival. Pocket Books, New York NY, 2000

[276] Isaacs, Scott, Hormonal Balance, Understanding Hormones, Weight, and Your Metabolism. Bull Publishing, Boulder, Colorado. 2002. P.3

[277] Traish AM, Saad F, Guay A. The Dark Side of Testosterone Deficiency: II. Type 2 Diabetes and Insulin Resistance. J Androl. 2009 Jan-Feb;30(1):23-32.

[278] Leder BZ, Rohrer JL, et al. Effects of Aromatase Inhibition in Elderly Men With Low or Borderline-low Serum Testosterone Levels. J Clin Endocrinol Metab. 2004 Mar;89(3):1174-80.

[279] Lakshman KM, Basaria S. Safety and Efficacy of Testosterone Gel in the Treatment of Male Hypogonadism. Clin Interv Aging. 2009;4:397-412.

[280] Lee, John., What Your Doctor May Not Tell You About Premenopause. Warner Books. New York, New York. 1999; pp. 55-75.

[281] Bergkvist L, Adami H-O, Persson I, Hoover R, Schairer C. The Risk of Breast Cancer after Estrogen and Estrogen-progestin Replacement. N Eggl J Med 1989; 321:293-297.

[282] Chang KJ, Lee TTY, Linares-Cruz G, Fourinier S, de Lignieres B. Influences of Percutaneous Administration of Estradiol and Progesterone on Human Breast Epithelial Cell Cycle in Vivo. Fertility and Sterility 1995;63:785-791.

[283] Guyton, Arthur C. &Hall, John E., Textbook of Medical Physiology, 11th Edition; Saunders Publishing, 2005

[284] How To Get Your Cholesterol Tested. http://www.heart.org/HEARTORG/Conditions/Cholesterol/SymptomsDiagnosisMonitoringofHighCholesterol/How-To-Get-Your-Cholesterol-Tested_UCM_305595_Article.jsp

[285] Choices in Testing for Complete Cardiovascular Care, http://www.labcorp.com/pdf/Cardiovascular_flyer_L4719_0407_1.pdf

[286] Otvos JD. Measurement of Lipoprotein Subclass Profiles by Nuclear Magnetic Resonance Spectroscopy. In: Rifai N, Warnick GR, Dominiczak MH, eds. *Handbook of Lipoprotein Testing*. 2nd ed. Washington DC: AACC Press; 2000:609-623.

[287] Otvos J, Jeyarajah E, Bennett D. A Spectroscopic Approach to Lipoprotein Subclass Analysis. *J Clin Ligand Assay*. 1996; 19(3):184-189.

[288] VAP: The Most Comprehensive Cholesterol Test. http://www.atherotech.com/

[289] Genest JJ, McNamara JR, Salem DN, Schaefer EJ. Prevalence of Risk Factors in Men with Premature Coronary Artery Disease. *Am J Cardiol*. 1991; 67:1185-1189.

[290] Kannel WB. Range of Serum Cholesterol Values in the Population Developing Coronary Artery Disease. *Amer J Cardiol*. 1995; 76:69C-77C.

[291] Chatzizisis YS, Koskinas KC, et al. Risk Factors and Drug Interactions Predisposing to Statin-Induced Myopathy: Implications for Risk Assessment, Prevention and Treatment. Drug Saf. 2010 Mar 1;33(3):171-87.

[292] Schwartz GG, Olsson AG, Ezekowitz MD, et al. Effects of Atorvastatin on Early Recurrent Ischemic Events in Acute Coronary Syndromes. The MIRACL Study: A Randomized Controlled Trial. *JAMA*. 2001; 285(13):1711-1718.

[293] Rubins HB, Robins SJ, Collins D, et al. Gemfibrozil for the Secondary Prevention of Coronary Heart Disease in Men With Low Levels of High-Density Lipoprotein Cholesterol. The Veteran Affairs High-Density Lipoprotein Cholesterol Intervention Trial Study Group. *N Eng J Med*. 1999; 341(6):410-418.

[294] Miller DB. Secondary Prevention for Ischemic Heart Disease: Relative Numbers Needed to Treat with Different Therapies. *Arch IntMed*. 1997; 157:2045-2052.

[295] Ridker PM, Rifai N, Rose L, Buring JE, Cook NR. Comparison of C-Reactive Protein and Low-Density Lipoprotein Cholesterol Levels in the Prediction of First Cardiovascular Events. N Engl J Med 2002;347:1557-1565.

[296] Ridker PM, et al. C-Reactive Protein Levels and Outcomes after Statin Therapy. New England Journal of Medicine, Jan 6, 2005; 352: 20-28

[297] Winslow R. Heart-Disease Sleuths Identify Prime Suspect: Inflammation of Artery, *Wall Street Journal*, October 7, 1999

[298] Know Your Fats. American Heart Association Website; http://www.heart.org/HEARTORG/Conditions/Cholesterol/PreventionTreatmentof HighCholesterol/Know-Your-Fats_UCM_305628_Article.jsp

[299] What Causes Heart Disease? http://trit.us/moderndiseases/hd.html

[300] Mozaffarian D, Katan MB, Ascherio A, Stampfer MJ, Willett WC. Trans Fatty Acids and Cardiovascular Disease. *N Engl J Med*. 2006; 354:1601-13.

[301] Willett WC, Stampfer MJ, Manson JE, et al. Intake of Trans Fatty Acids and Risk of Coronary Heart Disease Among Women. *Lancet*. 1993; 341:581-585.

[302] Hu FB, Stampfer MJ, Rimm EB, et al. A Prospective Study of Egg Consumption and Risk of Cardiovascular Disease in Men and Women. *JAMA*. 1999; 281:1387-94.

[303] Fernandez ML. Dietary Cholesterol Provided by Eggs and Plasma Lipoproteins in Healthy Populations. *Curr Opin Clin Nutr Metab Care*. 2006; 9:8-12.

[304] Holvoet P, et al. The Metabolic Syndrome, Circulating Oxidized LDL, and Risk of Myocardial Infarction in Well-Functioning Elderly People in the Health, Aging, and Body Composition Cohort. Diabetes, Apr 1, 2004; 53(4): 1068-1073.

[305] Osterud B, Bjorklid E. Role of Monocytes in Atherogenesis. Physiol Rev. 2003 Oct;83(4):1069-112.

[306] Kristenson M, et al. Antioxidant State and Mortality from Coronary Heart Disease in Lithuanian and Swedish Men: Concomitant Cross Sectional Study of Men Aged 50. British Medical Journal, Mar, 1997; 314: 629.

[307] Matthias, B. and Schulze, M.B. Dietary Pattern, Inflammation, and Incidence of Type 2 Diabetes in Women. Am J Clin Nutr. Sep 2005; 82: 675-684.

[308] Heaton, K. The Sweet Road to Gallstones. Brit Med J. Apr 14, 1984; 288: 1103-1104.

[309] Welsh et al., Caloric Sweetener Consumption and Dyslipidemia Among US Adults, JAMA, April 2010, 303(15)

[310] Yudkin, J. Sugar Consumption and Myocardial Infarction. Lancet. Feb 6, 1971; 1(7693): 296-297.

[311] Profiling Food Consumption in America. http://www.usda.gov/factbook/chapter2.pdf

[312] Enig, Mary G, PhD, *Trans Fatty Acids in the Food Supply: A Comprehensive Report Covering 60 Years of Research*, 2nd Edition, Enig Associates, Inc, Silver Spring, MD, 1995, 4-8

[313] Fernandez, N A, *Cancer Res*, 1975, 35:3272; Martines, I, et al, Cancer Res, 1975, 35:3265

[314] Pitskhelauri, G Z, *The Long Living of Soviet Georgia*, 1982, Human Sciences Press, New York, NY

[315] Koga, Y et al, "Recent Trends in Cardiovascular Disease and Risk Factors in the Seven Countries Study: Japan," *Lessons for Science from the Seven Countries Study*, H Toshima, et al, eds, Springer, New York, NY, 1994, 63-74

[316] Moore, Thomas J, *Lifespan: What Really Affects Human Longevity*, 1990, Simon and Schuster, New York, NY

[317] Enig, Mary G, Ph D, et al, *Fed Proc*, Jul 1978, 37:9:2215-2220

[318] How Does Your Heart Function? http://www.besthearthealth.com/about.html

[319] Guyton, Arthur C. &Hall, John E., Textbook of Medical Physiology, 11th Edition; Saunders Publishing, 2005

[320] ibid

[321] Akay S, Ozdemir M. Acute Coronary Syndrome Presenting After Pseudoephedrine Use and Regression with Beta-Blocker Therapy. Can J Cardiol. 2008 Nov;24(11):e86-8.

[322] Cherry DK, Woodwell DA. National Ambulatory Medical Care Survey: 2000 Summary. *Advance Data.* 2002;328.

[323] Hypertension. http://www.cdc.gov/nchs/fastats/hyprtens.htm

[324] Antihypertensive Medication Use Among US Adults with Hypertension Qiuping Gu, Ryne Paulose-Ram, et al. Circulation. 2006;113:213-221

[325] National High Blood Pressure Education Program. http://www.nhlbi.nih.gov/guidelines/hypertension/express.pdf

[326] Heijer T, et al. Homocysteine and Brain Atrophy on MRI of Non-demented Elderly. Brain. 2002;1:170-175

[327] Van Den Kommer TN, Dik MG, et al. Homocysteine and Inflammation: Predictors of Cognitive Decline in Older Persons? Neurobiol Aging. 2008 Nov 10.

[328] Oudi ME, Aouni Z, et al. Homocysteine and Markers of Inflammation in Acute Coronary Syndrome. Exp Clin Cardiol. 2010 Summer;15(2):e25-8.

[329] Saposnik G, Ray JG, et al. Homocysteine-Lowering Therapy and Stroke Risk, Severity, and Disability: Additional Findings from the HOPE 2 Trial. Stroke. 2009 Apr;40(4):1365-72.

[330] Yilmaz N, Pektas M, et al. The Correlation of Plasma Homocysteine with Insulin Resistance in Polycystic Ovary Syndrome. J Obstet Gynaecol Res. 2008 Jun;34(3):384-91.

[331] Hirsch S, Poniachick J, et al. Serum Folate and Homocysteine Levels in Obese Females with Non-alcoholic Aatty Liver. Nutrition. 2005 Feb;21(2):137-41.

[332] Prasad AS, Lei KY, et al. Effect of Oral Contraceptives on Nutrients. III. Vitamins B6, B12, and Folic Acid. *Am J Obstet Gynecol.* 1976 Aug 15;125(8):1063-9.

[333] A Healthy Thyroid, http://www.aace. com/public/ awareness/tam/2005/pdfs/thyroid_disease_fact_sheet.pdf American Academy of Clinical Endocrinologists.

[334] Brownstein, David. Overcoming Thyroid Disorders. Medical Alternative Press, West Bloomfield MI, 2004. P. 51

[335] Pansini, F., et al. Effect of Hormonal Contraception on Serum Reverse Triiodothyronie Levels. Gynecol. Obstet. Invest., 23:133. 1987

[336] Kharrazain, Datis. Why do I Still Have Thyroid Symptoms When my Lab Tests are Normal? Morgan James Publishing. Garden City, New York; 2010

[337] Canaris GJ, Manowitz NR, Mayor G. The Colorado Thyroid Disease Prevalence Study. *Arch Intern Med.* Feb 28 2000;160(4):526-34.

[338] Bailleres. Autoimmunity and Hypothyroidism. *Clin Endocrin Metab.* 1988 Aug;2(3):591-617.

[339] Eur J Endocrinol. 2004 Mar; 150(3):363-9

[340] Neuro Endocrinol Lett. 2006 Aug 5;27

[341] Thyroid Antibodies. www.labtestsonline.org

[342] Kharrazain, Datis. Why do I Still Have Thyroid Symptoms When my Lab Tests are Normal? Morgan James Publishing. Garden City, New York; 2010

[343] ibid

[344] Mainardi E, Montanelli A, et al. Thyroid-related Autoantibodies and Celiac Disease: A Role for a Gluten-free Diet? *J Clin Gastroenterol.* 2002 Sep;35(3):245-8.

[345] Ch'ng CL, Jones MK, Kingham JG. Celiac Disease and Autoimmune Thyroid Disease. *Clin Med Res.* 2007 Oct;5(3):184-92.

[346] Iuorio R, Mercuri V, et al. Prevalence of Celiac Disease in Patients with Autoimmune Thyroiditis. *Minerva Endocrinol.* 2007 Dec;32(4):239-43.

[347] Kharrazain, Datis. Why do I Still Have Thyroid Symptoms When my Lab Tests are Normal? Morgan James Publishing. Garden City, New York; 2010, p. 27

[348] Ibid. pp.224-225

[349] Holick MF. Sunlight and Vitamin D for Bone Health and the Prevention of Autoimmune Diseases, Cancers and Cardiovascular Diseases. *Am J Clin Nutr* 2004:80:1678S-1688S.

[350] Buford TW, Willoughby DS. Impact of DHEA(S) and Cortisol on Immune Function in Aging: A Brief Review. Appl Physiol Nutr Metab. 2008 Jun;33(3):429-33.

[351] Fontana L. Neuroendocrine Factors in the Regulation of Inflammation: Excessive Adiposity and Calorie Restriction. Exp Gerontol. 2009 Jan-Feb;44(1-2):41-5.

[352] Van Santen A, Vreeburg SA, et al. Psychological Traits and the Cortisol Awakening Response: Results from the Netherlands Study of Depression and Anxiety. Psychoneuroendocrinology. 2010 Aug 17.

[353] Mujica-Parodi LR, Renelique R, Taylor MK. Higher Body Fat Percentage is Associated with Increased Cortisol Reactivity and Impaired Cognitive Resilience in Response to Acute Emotional Stress. Int J Obes (Lond). 2009 Jan;33(1):157-65.

[354] Gill RE, Hirst EL, Jones JK. Constitution of the Mucilage from the Bark of Ulmus Fulva (slippery elm mucilage); the Sugars Formed in the Hydrolysis of the Methylated Mucilage. J Chem Soc. 1946 Nov:1025-9.

[355] Deters A, Zippel J, Hellenbrand N, Pappai D, Possemeyer C, Hensel A. Aqueous Extracts and Polysaccharides from Marshmallow roots (Althea offi cinalis L.): cellular Internalisation and Stimulation of Cell Physiology of Human Epithelial Cells in Vitro. J Ethnopharmacol. 2010 Jan 8;127(1):62-9.

[356] Marks IN, Boyd E. Mucosal Protective Agents in the Long-Term Management of Gastric Ulcer. Med J Aust. 1985 Feb 4;142(3):S23-5.

[357] Food Allergies. http://www.cdc.gov/healthyyouth/foodallergies/

[358] Landau, Elizabeth. Why are Food Allergies on the Rise? http://www.cnn.com/2010/HEALTH/08/03/food.allergies.er.gut/?hpt=C2

[359] US Food and Drug Administration. Food Allergies: What You Need to Know.http://www.fda.gov/Food/ResourcesForYou/Consumers/ucm079311.htm.

[360] Turnbull, JA. "Changes in Sensitivity to Allergenic Foods in Arthritis." Am J. Dig. Dis 1994; 11:182

[361] Brownstein, David. Overcoming Arthritis. Medical Alternative Press, West Bloomfield MI, 2001. P. 141

[362] Nambudripad Allergy Elimination Technique; http://www.naet.com

[363] BioSet; http://www.drellencutler.com

[364] Nambudripad, Devi. Say Goodbye To Your Allergies. 2003

[365] Brimhall, John. Six Steps to Wellness. http://www.brimhallwellness center.com

[366] Cutler, Ellen. Live Free from Asthma and Allergies: Use the BioSET System to Detoxify and Desensitize Your Body. Celestial Arts, Berkeley CA; 2007.

[367] Pellicano R, Peyre S, et al. Updated Review on Helicobacter Pylori as a Potential Target for the Therapy of Ischemic Heart Disease (2006). Panminerva Med. 2006 Dec;48(4):241-6.

[368] Pellicano R, Parravicini PP, et al. Infection by Helicobacter Pylori and Acute Myocardial Infarction. Do Cytotoxic Strains Make a Difference? New Microbiol. 2002 Jul;25(3):315-21.

[369] Kharrazain, Datis. Why do I Still Have Thyroid Symptoms When my Lab Tests Are Normal? Morgan James Publishing. Garden City, New York; 2010

[370] Diamant M, Blaak EE, de Vos WM. Do Nutrient-Gut-Microbiota Interactions Play a Role in Human Obesity, Insulin Resistance and Type 2 Diabetes? Obes Rev. 2010 Aug 13.

[371] Neyrinck AM, Delzenne NM. Potential Interest of Gut Microbial Changes Induced by Non-Digestible Carbohydrates of Wheat in the Management of Obesity and Related Disorders. Curr Opin Clin Nutr Metab Care. 2010 Sep 4.

[372] Brownstein, David. Overcoming Arthritis. Medical Alternative Press, West Bloomfield MI, 2001. P. 13

[373] Subramanya D, Grivas PD. HPV and Cervical Cancer: Updates on an Established Relationship. Postgrad Med. 2008 Nov;120(4):7-13.

[374] Lawson JS. Do Viruses Cause Breast Cancer? Methods Mol Biol. 2009;471:421-38.

[375] Sauce D, Larsen M, et al. EBV-Associated Mononucleosis Leads to Long-Term Global Deficit in T-cell Responsiveness to IL-15. Blood. 2006 Jul 1;108(1):11-8.

[376] Am J Public Health. 2004 May; 94(5): 746–747.

[377] James M. Perrin, MD; Sheila R. Bloom, MS; Steven L. Gortmaker, PhD The Increase of Childhood Chronic Conditions in the United States. JAMA. 2007;297:2755-2759.

[378] Zimm, Angela. Children Sicker Now Than in Past, Harvard Report Says. http://www.bloomberg.com

[379] American Autoimmune Related Diseases Association, Inc.

[380] Jacobson DL et al. Clin Immunol Immunopathol, 84: 223-243, 1997

[381] Fitch E, Harper E, et al. Pathophysiology of Psoriasis: Recent Advances on IL-23 and Th17 Cytokines. Curr Rheumatol Rep. 2007 Dec;9(6):461-7.

[382] Brownstein, David. Overcoming Arthritis. Medical Alternative Press, West Bloomfield MI, 2001. P. 154

[383] Batmanghelidj, F. Your Body's Many Cries for Water. http://www.watercure.com/

[384] Migraine. http://www.womenshealth.gov/faq/migraine.cfm#b

[385] ibid

[386] Edlow AG, Bartz D. Hormonal Contraceptive Options for Women with Headache: A Review of the Evidence. Rev Obstet Gynecol. 2010 Spring;3(2):55-65.

[387] Wirth JJ, Mijal RS. Adverse Effects of Low Level Heavy Metal Exposure on Male Reproductive Function. Syst Biol Reprod Med. 2010 Apr;56(2):147-67.

[388] Iavicoli I, Fontana L, Bergamaschi A. The Effects of Metals as Endocrine Disruptors. J Toxicol Environ Health B Crit Rev. 2009 Mar;12(3):206-23.

[389] Houston MC. The Role of Mercury and Cadmium Heavy Metals in Vascular Disease, Hypertension, Coronary Heart Disease, and Myocardial Infarction. Altern Ther Health Med. 2007 Mar-Apr;13(2):S128-33.

[390] Walton JR.. Evidence for Participation of Aluminum in Neurofibrillary Tangle Formation and Growth in Alzheimer's Disease. J Alzheimers Dis. 2010 Aug 30.

[391] Monnet-Tschudi F, Zurich MG, et al. Involvement of Environmental Mercury and Lead in the Etiology of Neurodegenerative Diseases. Rev Environ Health. 2006 Apr Jun;21(2):105-17.

[392] McGoey, B. V., Deitel, M., Saplys, R. J., Kliman, M. E. (1990) Effect of Weight Loss on Musculoskeletal Pain in the Morbidly Obese. J Bone Joint Surg 72: 322–323.

[393] Fontaine, K. R., Barofsky, I., Andersen, R. E., et al. (1999) Impact of Weight Loss on Health-related Quality of Life. Qual Life Res 8: 275–277.

[394] Williamson, D. F., Pamuk, E., Thun, M., Flanders, D., Byers, T., Heath, C. (1999) Prospective Study of Intentional Weight Loss and Mortality in Overweight White Women Aged 40 – 64 Years. Am J Epidemiol 149: 491–503.

[395] Mozaffarian D, Rimm EB. Fish Intake, Contaminants, and Human Health: Evaluating the Risks and the Benefits. JAMA. 2006; 296:1885-99.

[396] ibid

[397] Järup L. Hazards of Heavy Metal Contamination. Br Med Bull. 2003;68:167-82.

[398] Galal-Gorchev H. Food Addit Contam. Dietary Intake, Levels in Food and Estimated Intake of Lead, Cadmium, and Mercury. 1993 Jan-Feb;10(1):115-28.

[399] González-Weller D, Karlsson L, et al. Lead and Cadmium in Meat and Meat Products Consumed by the Population in Tenerife Island, Spain. Food Addit Contam. 2006 Aug;23(8):757-63.

[400] Järup L. Hazards of Heavy Metal Contamination. Br Med Bull. 2003;68:167-82.

[401] Brownstein, David. Overcoming Thyroid Disorders. Medical Alternative Press, West Bloomfield MI, 2004. P. 216-222

[402] Bosboom JL, Stoffers D, Wolters ECh. The Role of Acetylcholine and Dopamine in Dementia and Psychosis in Parkinson's Disease. J Neural Transm Suppl. 2003;(65):185-95.

[403] Hasselmo ME. The Role of Acetylcholine in Learning and Memory. Curr Opin Neurobiol. 2006 Dec;16(6):710-5. Epub 2006 Sep 29.

[404] Haense C, Kalbe E, et al. Cholinergic System Function and Cognition in Mild Cognitive Impairment. Neurobiol Aging. 2010 Oct 18.

[405] Resende RR, Adhikari A. Cholinergic Receptor Pathways Involved in Apoptosis, Cell Proliferation and Neuronal Differentiation. Cell Commun Signal. 2009 Aug 27;7:20.

[406] Skvortsova RI, Pzniakovski VM, Agarkova IA. Role of Vitamin Factor in Preventing Phenol Poisoning. Vopr Pitan 1981; 2: 32-35.

[407] Schrauzer G. Lithium Occurrences, Dietary Intakes, Nutritional Essentiality. JACN 2002; 21(1):14-21.

[408] Vanyo L, Vu T, et al. Lithium Induced Perturbations of Vitamin B12, Folic acid and DNA metabolism. In Schrauzer Gn, Klippel, KF(eds): Lithium in Biology and Medicine. Weinheim:VCH Verlag, pp 17-30, 1991.

[409] Spagnolie A, et al. Long-term Acetyl-L-carnitine Treatment in Alzheimer's Disease. Neurology 1991;41:1726-1732.

[410] Brownstein, David. Overcoming Thyroid Disorders. Medical Alternative Press, West Bloomfield MI, 2004. P. 187

[411] Yokosuka M, Ohtani-Kaneko R, et al. Estrogen and Environmental Estrogenic Chemicals Exert Developmental Effects on Rat Hypothalamic Neurons and Glias. Toxicol In Vitro. 2008 Feb;22(1):1-9.

[412] Min J, Lee SK, Gu MB. Effects of Endocrine Disrupting Chemicals on Distinct Expression Patterns of Estrogen Receptor, Cytochrome P450 aromatase and p53 genes in Oryzias Latipes Liver. J Biochem Mol Toxicol. 2003;17(5):272-7.

[413] Elliott Johansen, Bruce. The Dirty Dozen: Toxic Chemicals and Earth's Future. Praeger Publishers; 2003. P. 150

[414] Sánchez-Pernaute O, Ospelt C, Neidhart M, Gay S. Epigenetic Clues to Rheumatoid Arthritis. J Autoimmun. 2008 Feb-Mar;30(1-2):12-20. Epub 2007 Dec 26.

[415] Wilson AG. Epigenetic Regulation of Gene Expression in the Inflammatory Response and Relevance to Common Diseases. J Periodontol. 2008 Aug;79(8 Suppl):1514-9.

[416] Campbell TC, Chen JS, Liu CB, Li JY, Parpia B. Nonassociation of Aflatoxin With Primary Liver Cancer in a Cross-Sectional Ecological Survey in the People's Republic of China. Cancer Res. 1990 Nov 1;50(21):6882-93.

[417] Sudakin DL. Dietary Aflatoxin Exposure and Chemoprevention of Cancer: A Clinical Review. J Toxicol Clin Toxicol. 2003;41(2):195-204.

[418] Patten RC. Aflatoxins and Disease. Am J Trop Med Hyg. 1981 Mar;30(2):422-5.

[419] Podas T, Nightingale JM, et al. Is Rheumatoid Arthritis a Disease that Starts in the Intestine? Postgrad Med J. 2007 Feb;83(976):128-31.

[420] Koboziev I, Karlsson F, Grisham MB. Gut-Associated Lymphoid Tissue, T cell Trafficking, and Chronic Intestinal Inflammation.
Ann N Y Acad Sci. 2010 Oct;1207

[421] Brownstein, David. Overcoming Arthritis. Medical Alternative Press, West Bloomfield MI, 2001. P. 13

[422] Nicklas RA. Sulfites: A Review With Emphasis on Biochemistry and Clinical Application. Allergy Proc. 1989 Sep-Oct;10(5):349-56.

[423] Yang WH, Purchase EC. Adverse Reactions to Sulfites. CMAJ. 1985 Nov 1;133(9):865-7, 880.

[424] Antonovsky, A. "Health, Stress and Coping" San Francisco: Jossey-Bass Publishers, 1979

[425] Antonovsky, A. Unraveling The Mystery of Health - How People Manage Stress and Stay Well, San Francisco: Jossey-Bass Publishers, 1987

[426] Esch T, Stefano GB. The Neurobiology of Pleasure, Reward Processes, Addiction and their Health Implications. Neuro Endocrinol Lett. 2004 Aug;25(4):235-51.

[427] Dawson R Jr., Pelleymounter MA, Cullen NJ, Gollub M, Liu S. "An Age Related Decline in Striatal Taurine is Correlated With a Loss of Dopaminergic Markers." Brain Res Bull 1999 Feb; 48(3); 319-24.

[428] Bosboom JL, Stoffers D, Wolters ECh. The Role of Acetylcholine and Dopamine in Dementia and Psychosis in Parkinson's disease. J Neural Transm Suppl. 2003;(65):185-95.

[429] Volz TJ. Neuropharmacological Mechanisms Underlying the Neuroprotective Effects of Methylphenidate [Ritalin].

[430] Rate of Parent-Reported ADHD Increasing.
http://www.cdc.gov/ncbddd/features/adhd-parent-reporting.html

[431] Colter AL, Cutler C, Meckling KA. Fatty Acid Status and Behavioral Symptoms of Attention Deficit Hyperactivity
Disorder in Adolescents: A Case-Control Study. Nutr J. 2008 Feb 14;7:8.

[432] Stevens LJ, Zentall SS, Deck JL, Abate ML, Watkins BA, Lipp SR, Burgess JR. Essential Fatty Acid Metabolism in Boys with Attention-Deficit Hyperactivity Disorder. Am J Clin Nutr. 1995 Oct;62(4):761-8.

[433] Burgess JR, Stevens L, Zhang W, Peck L. Long-Chain Polyunsaturated Fatty Acids in Children with Attention-Deficit Hyperactivity Disorder. Am J Clin Nutr. 2000 Jan;71(1 Suppl):327S-30S.

[434] Dodig-Curković K, et al. The Role of Zinc in the Treatment of Hyperactivity Disorder in Children. Acta Med Croatica. 2009 Oct;63(4):307-13.

[435] Guilarate TR. Effects of Vitamin B-6 Nutrition on the Levels of Dopamine, Dopamine Metabolites, Dopa Decarboxylase Activity, Tyrosine, and GABA in the Developing Rat Corpus Striatum. Neurochemical Research 1989;14:571-578.

[436] Harmer CJ, McTavish SF, Clark L, Goodwin GM, Cowen PJ. Tyrosine

Depletion Attenuates Dopamine Function in Healthy Volunteers.
Psychopharmacology (Berl). 2001;154(1):105-11.

[437] Huss M, Völp A, Stauss-Grabo M. Supplementation of Polyunsaturated Fatty Acids, Magnesium and Zinc in Children Seeking Medical Advice for Attention-Deficit/Hyperactivity Problems – An Observational Cohort Study. Lipids Health Dis. 2010 Sep 24;9:105.

[438] Rucklidge JJ, Johnstone J, Kaplan BJ. Nutrient Supplementation Approaches in the Treatment of ADHD. Expert Rev Neurother. 2009 Apr;9(4):461-76.

[439] Cruz NV, Bahna SL. Do Food or Additives Cause Behavior Disorders? Pediatr Ann. 2006 Oct;35(10):744-5, 748-54.

[440] Sinn N. Nutritional and Dietary Influences on Attention Deficit Hyperactivity Disorder. Nutr Rev. 2008 Oct;66(10):558-68.

[441] Maier SF, Watkins LR. Cytokines for Psychologists: Implications of Bidirectional Immune-to-Brain Communication for Understanding Behavior, Mood, and Cognition. Psychol Rev. 1998 Jan;105(1):83-107.

[442] Audet MC, Mangano EN, Anisman H. Behavior and Pro-Inflammatory Cytokine Variations among Submissive and Dominant Mice Engaged in Aggressive Encounters: Moderation by Corticosterone Reactivity. Front Behav Neurosci. 2010 Aug 23;4. pii: 156.

[443] Covelli V, Passeri ME, Leogrande D, Jirillo E, Amati L. Drug Targets in Stress-Related Disorders. Curr Med Chem. 2005;12(15):1801-9 | PMID:16029148

[444] http://www.909shot.com

[445] Dodig-Curković K, et al. The Role of Zinc in the Treatment of Hyperactivity Disorder in Children. Acta Med Croatica. 2009 Oct;63(4):307-13.

[446] Volz TJ. Neuropharmacological Mechanisms Underlying the Neuroprotective Effects of Methylphenidate [Ritalin].
Curr Neuropharmacol. 2008 Dec;6(4):379-85.

[447] Plassman BL, et al. Prevalence of Dementia in the United States: The Aging, Demographics, and Memory Study. Neuroepidemiology. 2007;29(1-2):125-32.

[448] Plassman BL, et al. Prevalence of Dementia in the United States: The Aging, Demographics, and Memory Study. Neuroepidemiology. 2007;29(1-2):125-32.

[449] Bosboom JL, Stoffers D, Wolters ECh. The Role of Acetylcholine and Dopamine in Dementia and Psychosis in Parkinson's disease. J Neural Transm Suppl. 2003;(65):185-95.

[450] Walton JR. Evidence for Participation of Aluminum in Neurofibrillary Tangle Formation and Growth in Alzheimer's Disease.
J Alzheimers Dis. 2010 Aug 30.

[451] Monnet-Tschudi F, Zurich MG, et al. Involvement of Environmental Mercury and Lead in the Etiology of Neurodegenerative Diseases. Rev Environ Health. 2006 Apr Jun;21(2):105-17.

[452] Lee PH, Yong SW, An YS. Changes in Cerebral Glucose Metabolism in Patients with Parkinson Disease with Dementia after Cholinesterase Inhibitor Therapy. J Nucl Med. 2008 Dec;49(12):2006-11. Epub 2008 Nov 7.

[453] Hasselmo ME. The Role of Acetylcholine in Learning and Memory. Curr Opin Neurobiol. 2006 Dec;16(6):710-5.

[454] Hasselmo ME, Sarter M. Modes and Models of Forebrain Cholinergic Neuromodulation of Cognition. Neuropsychopharmacology. 2011 Jan;36(1):52-73.

[455] Jin CY, Lee JD, Park C, Choi YH, Kim GY. Curcumin Attenuates the Release of Pro-Inflammatory Cytokines in Lipoplysaccharide-Stimulated BV2 Microglia.ActaPharmacol Sin. 2007;28(10):1645-51.

[456] Jin CY, Lee JD, Park C, Choi YH, Kim GY. Curcumin Attenuates the Release of Pro-Inflammatory Cytokines in Lipoplysaccharide-Stimulated BV2 Microglia.ActaPharmacol Sin. 2007;28(10):1645-51.

[457] Huang O, Wu LJ, Tashiro S, Onedera S, Ikejima T. Elevated levels of DNA Repair Enzymes and Antioxidative Enzymes by (+)-Catechin in Murinemicroglia Cells after Oxidative Stress. J Asian Nat Prod Res. 8(1-2):61-71.

[458] Rezai-Zaldeh K, Ehrhart J, Bai Y, Sansberg PR, Bickfored P, Tan J, ShytelD. Apigenin and Luteolin Modulate Microglial Activation via Inhibition of STAT-1 Induced CD40 Expression. J Neuroinflammation. 2008;25(5):41.

[459] Chen HO, Jin ZY, Wang XJ, Xu XM, Deng L, Zhao JW. Luteolin Protects Dopaminergic Neurons from Inflammation-Induced Injury through Inhibitionof Microglial Activation. NeurosciLett. 2008;448(2):175-179.

[460] Suk K, Lee H, Kang SS, CHO GJ, Choi WS. Flavonoid Baicalein Attenuates Activation-induced Cell Death of Brain Microglia. J Pharmacol ExpTher. 2003;305(2):638-45.

[461] Iacoboni, Marco. *Mirroring People*. Farrar, Straus and Giroux, 2008.

[462] Klingberg T. Training and Plasticity of Working Memory. Trends Cogn Sci. 2010 Jul;14(7):317-24.

[463] Baddeley A. Working Memory. Science. 1992 Jan 31;255(5044):556-9.

[464] McNab F, Varrone A, et al. Science. Changes in Cortical Dopamine D1 Receptor Binding Associated With Cognitive Training. 2009 Feb 6;323(5915):800-2.

[465] McNab F, Klingberg T. Prefrontal Cortex and Basal Ganglia Control Access to Working Memory. Nat Neurosci. 2008 Jan;11(1):103-7.

[466] Bingo 'Helps Beat Memory Loss', Ananova News Portal, February 23, 2001 http://www.ananova.com/news/story/sm_217474.html

[467] Sharot T, Shiner T, et al. Dopamine Enhances Expectation of Pleasure in Humans. Curr Biol. 2009 Dec 29;19(24):2077-80.

[468] Trenkwalder C, Seidel VC, Gasser T, Oertel WH. Clinical Symptoms and Possible anticipation in a Large Kindred of Familial Restless Legs Syndrome. Mov Disord 1996; 11:389-394

[469] Howes OD, Montgomery AJ, et al. Elevated Striatal Dopamine Function Linked to Prodromal Signs of Schizophrenia. Arch Gen Psychiatry. 2009 Jan;66(1):13-20.

[470] McGowan S, Lawrence AD, et al. Presynaptic Dopaminergic Dysfunction in Schizophrenia: A Positron Emission Tomographic [18F] Fluorodopa study. Arch Gen Psychiatry. 2004 Feb;61(2):134-42.

[471] Pitchot W, Hansenne M, Ansseau M. Role of Dopamine in Non-Depressed Patients with a History of Suicide Attempts. Eur Psychiatry. 2001 Nov;16(7):424-7.

[472] Guilleminault C, Palombini L, et al. Sleepwalking and Sleep Terrors in Prepubertal Children: What Triggers Them? Pediatrics. 2003 Jan;111(1):e17-25.

[473] Maton PN, Burton ME. Antacids Revisited: A Review of Their Clinical Pharmacology and Recommended Therapeutic Use.Drugs. 1999 Jun;57(6):855-70.

[474] Sontag SJ. The Medical Management of Reflux Esophagitis. Role of Antacids and Acid Inhibition. GastroenterolClin North Am. 1990 Sep;19(3):683-712.

[475] Ching CK, Lam SK. Antacids. Indications and Limitations. Drugs. 1994 Feb;47(2):305-17.

[476] Scarpignato C, Pelosini I, Di Mario F. Acid Suppression Therapy: Where Do We Go From Here? Dig Dis. 2006;24(1-2):11-46.

[477] Guhad, FA, et al. Salivary IgA as a Marker of Social Stress in Rats. NeurosciLett,216(2). 137-140,1996.

[478] Evans MA and Shronts EP. Intestinal Fuels: Glutamine, Short-chain Fatty Acids, and Dietary Fiber. J Amer Diet Assoc 92, 1239-1246,1992.

[479] http://www.cdc.gov/ulcer/files/hpfacts.PDF

[480] Eidt S, Stolte M. The Significance of Helicobacter Pylori in Relation to Gastric Cancer and Lymphoma.Eur J GastroenterolHepatol. 1995 Apr;7(4):318-21.

[481] Cheon JH, Kim JH, et al. Helicobacter Pylori Eradication Therapy May Facilitate Gastric Ulcer Healing after Endoscopic Mucosal Resection: A Prospective Randomized Study. Helicobacter. 2008 Dec;13(6):564-71.

[482] Hunt, RH. *Helicobacter Pylori*: from Theory to Practice. Proceedings of a Symposium. Am J Med1996; 100 (5A) supplement.

[483] Kowalski M, Pawlik M, et al. Helicobacter Pylori Infection in Coronary Artery Disease. J PhysiolPharmacol. 2006 Sep;57Suppl 3:101-11.

[484] http://www.cdc.gov/ulcer/files/hpfacts.PDF

[485] Hobsley M, Tovey FI, Holton J. Controversies in the Helicobacter Pylori/Duodenal Ulcer Story.Trans R Soc Trop Med Hyg. 2008 Dec;102(12):1171-5. Epub 2008 Jun 26.

[486] Beil W, Birkholz, Sewing KF. Effects of Flavonoids on Parietal Cell Acid Secretion, Gastric Mucosal Prostaglandin Production and Helicobacter Pylori Growth.ArzeneimForsch. 1995;45:697-700.

[487] Marle J, et al. Deglycrrhizinated Liquorice (DGL) and the Renewal of Rat Stomachepithelium. Eur J Pharm 1981;72:219.

[488]11Kang Jy, et al. Effect of Colloidal Bismuth Subcitrate on Symptoms and Gastrichistology in Non-ulcer Dyspepsia. A Double Blind Placebo Controlled Study. Gut.1990;31: 476-480.

[489] Rich P. Cutis. Hormonal Contraceptives for Acne Management. 2008 Jan;81(1 Suppl):13-8.

[490]Kimball AB. Advances in the Treatment of Acne. J Reprod Med. 2008 Sep;53(9 Suppl):742-52.

[491]Yosipovitch G, Tang M, et al. Study of Psychological Stress, Sebum Production and Acne Vulgaris in Adolescents. ActaDermVenereol. 2007;87(2):135-9.

[492]Chiu A, Chon SY, Kimball AB. The Response of Skin Disease to Stress: Changes in the Severity of Acne Vulgaris as Affected by Examination Stress. Arch Dermatol. 2003 Jul;139(7):897-900.

[493] Li YF, Jackson KL, et al. Interaction between Glutamate and GABA Systems in the Integration of Sympathetic Outflow by the Paraventricular Nucleus of the Hypothalamus. Am J Physiol Heart Circ Physiol. 2006 Dec;291(6):H2847-56.

[494]Kiani, Leila. Bugs in Our Guts. http://www.csa.com/discoveryguides/ probiotic/review.pdf

[495] Romeo J, Nova E, et al. Immunomodulatory Effect of Fibres, Probiotics and Synbiotics in Different Life-Stages. Nutr Hosp. 2010 May-Jun;25(3):341-9.

[496]Gourbeyre P, Denery S, Bodinier M. Probiotics, Prebiotics, and Synbiotics: Impact on the Gut Immune System and Allergic Reactions. J Leukoc Biol. 2011 Jan 13.

[497]Moayyedi P, Ford AC, et al. The Efficacy of Probiotics in the Treatment of Irritable Bowel Syndrome: A Systematic Review. Gut. 2010 Mar;59(3):325-32.

[498] Del Piano M, Carmagnola S, et al. The Use of Probiotics in Healthy Volunteers with Evacuation Disorders and Hard Stools: A Double-Blind, Randomized, Placebo-Controlled Study. J ClinGastroenterol. 2010 Sep;44Suppl 1:S30-4.

[499]Santos F, Vera JL, et al. The Complete Coenzyme B12 Biosynthesis Gene Cluster of Lactobacillus Reuteri CRL1098.Microbiology. 2008 Jan;154(Pt 1):81-93.

[500] http://digestive.niddk.nih.gov/ddiseases/pubs/constipation/index.htm

[501] Di Lorenzo C, Youssef NN. Diagnosis and Management of Intestinal Motility Disorders. SeminPediatr Surg. 2010 Feb;19(1):50-8.

[502]Ekanem AP, Brisibe EA. Effects of Ethanol Extract of Artemisia Annua L. AgainstMonogenean Parasites of Heterobranchus Longifilis. Parasitol Res. 2010 Apr;106(5):1135-9.

[503] Belknap JK. Black Walnut Extract: An Inflammatory Model. Vet Clin North Am Equine Pract. 2010 Apr;26(1):95-101.

[504] http://supremenutritionproducts.com/GoldenThreadSupreme/index.html

[505]Asthma. http://www.cdc.gov/nchs/fastats/asthma.htm

[506]Akinbami LJ, Schoendorf KC. Trends in Childhood Asthma: Prevalence, Health Care Utilization, and Mortality. Pediatrics 110 (2 Pt 1) :315–22. 2002.

[507] Rate of Parent-Reported ADHD Increasing.
http://www.cdc.gov/ncbddd/features/adhd-parent-reporting.html

[508] Zimm, Angela. Children Sicker Now Than in Past, Harvard Report Says.
http://www.bloomberg.com

[509] Lu WY, Inman MD. Gama-Aminobutyric Acid Nurtures Allergic Asthma. ClinExp Allergy. 2009 Jul;39(7):956-61.

[510] Xiang YY, Wang S, et al. A GABAergic System in Airway Epithelium is Essential for Mucus Overproduction in Asthma. Nat Med. 2007 Jul;13(7):862-7.

[511] McCormick DA. GABA as an Inhibitory Neurotransmitter in Human Cerebral Cortex.J Neurophysiol. 1989 Nov;62(5):1018-27.

[512] U.S. Department of Health and Human Services. (2003). National Survey of Child and Adolescent Well-Being: One Year in Foster Care Wave 1 Data Analysis Report. Retrieved April 27, 2006, from
www.acf.hhs.gov/programs/opre/abuse_neglect/nscaw/reports/nscaw_oyfc/oyfc_title.html

[513] Kelley, B. T., Thornberry, T. P., & Smith, C. A. (1997).In the Wake of Childhood Maltreatment. Washington, DC: National Institute of Justice. Retrieved April 27, 2006

[514] English, D. J., Widom, C. S., & Brandford, C. (2004). Another Look at the Effects of Child Abuse.NIJ journal, 251, 23-24.

[515] Long-Term Consequences of Child Abuse and Neglect
www.childwelfare.gov/pubs/factsheets/long_term_consequences.cfm#societ

[516] Craig, Gary. http://www.selfgrowth.com/experts/gary_craig.html

[517] Walker, Scott. http://www.netmindbody.com/net

[518] Callahan, R.J. and Callahan, J. (2000). Stop the Nightmares of Trauma. Chapel Hill: Professional Press. p. 143

[519] Ratey, John.Spark - The Revolutionary New Science of Exercise and the Brain. Little, Brown and Company; New York, NY 2008, p.236

[520] Pedersen BK, Akerström TC, et al. Role of Myokines in Exercise and Metabolism. J Appl Physiol. 2007 Sep;103(3):1093-8.

[521] Nielsen S, Pedersen BK. Skeletal Muscle as an Immunogenic Organ. CurrOpinPharmacol. 2008 Jun;8(3):346-51.

[522] Pedersen BK, Febbraio MA. Muscle as an Endocrine Organ: Focus on Muscle-Derived Interleukin-6. Physiol Rev. 2008 Oct;88(4):1379-406.

[523] Cao H, Gerhold K, et al. Identification of a Lipokine, a Lipid Hormone Linking Adipose Tissue to Systemic Metabolism. Cell. 2008 Sep 19;134(6):933-44.

[524] Wiley TS, Lights Out, Sleep Sugar and Survival. Pocket Books, New York NY, 2000; p. 94.

[525] La Gerche A, Prior DL. Exercise—Is it Possible to Have Too Much of a Good Thing? Heart Lung Circ. 2007;16Suppl 3:S102-4.

[526] Exercise and Acute Cardiovascular Events: Placing the Risks into Perspective.MedSci Sports Exerc. 2007 May;39(5):886-97.

[527]Wortsman.Role of Epinephrine in Acute Stress. J. EndocrinolMetabClin North Am. 2002 Mar;31(1):79-106.

[528]http://www.cdc.gov/vitalsigns/AdultObesity/index.html

[529]http://www.mypyramid.gov/STEPS/stepstoahealthierweight.html

INDEX

C

Bio Consulting & Education
Bio Energetic - Consulting Education
        Consulting and education
    Body Mind Spirit
    Bio-Etheric Health, —
Bioscience report levous
(structure + between +
    consulting +
        Educator, Inc

CPSIA information can be obtained at www.ICGtesting.com
Printed in the USA
BVOW081202280911

272347BV00003B/6/P